Vocational Rehabilitation and Europe

The Disability and Rehabilitation Series

Approaches to Case Management for People with Disabilities
Doria Pilling
ISBN 1 85302 099 0
Disability and Rehabilitation Series 1

Managing Disability at Work
Improving Practice in Organisations
Brenda Smith, Margary Povall and Michael Floyd
ISBN 1 85302 123 7
Disability and Rehabilitation Series 2

Information Technology Training for People with Disabilities
Edited by Michael Floyd
ISBN 1 85302 129 6
Disability and Rehabilitation Series 4

Mental Health at Work
Issues and Initiatives
Edited by Michael Floyd, Margery Povall and Graham Watson
ISBN 1 85302 177 6
Disability and Rehabilitation Series 5

Evaluating Quality in Services for Disabled and Older People
Edited by Doria Pilling and Graham Watson
ISBN 1 85302 289 6
Disability and Rehabilitation Series 7

Vocational Rehabilitation and Europe

Edited by Michael Floyd

Disability and Rehabilitation 6

Jessica Kingsley Publishers The Rehabilitation Resource Centre
London and Bristol, Pennsylvania London

All rights reserved. No paragraph of this publication may be reproduced, copied or transmitted save with written permission or in accordance with the provisions of the Copyright Act 1956 (as amended), or under the terms of any licence permitting limited copying issued by the Copyright Licensing Agency, 33–34 Alfred Place, London WC1E 7DP. Any person who does any unauthorised act in relation to this publication may be liable to criminal prosecution and civil claims for damages.

The right of the contributors to be identified as author of this work has been asserted by them in accordance with the Copyright, Designs and Patents Act 1988.

First published in the United Kingdom in 1997 by
Jessica Kingsley Publishers Ltd
116 Pentonville Road
London N1 9JB, England
and
1900 Frost Road, Suite 101
Bristol, PA 19007, U S A

and
The Rehabilitation Resource Centre
City University
Northampton Square
London EC1V 0HB

Copyright © 1997 the contributors and the Rehabilitation Resource Centre

Library of Congress Cataloging in Publication Data
Floyd, Michael, 1942–
Vocational rehabilitation and Europe / Michael Floyd.
p. cm. – (Disability and rehabilitation ; 6)
Includes bibliographical references (p.) and index.
ISBN 1-85302-235-7 (pb : alk paper)
1. Vocational rehabilitation – European Union countries.
2. Vocational rehabilitation – United States. 3. Vocational rehabilitation – Great Britain. I. Title II. Series: Disability and rehabilitation series ; 6.
HD7256.E9F58   1996
362'.0425–dc20   96-34235
                                                                    CIP

British Library Cataloguing in Publication Data
Vocational rehabilitation and Europe. - (Disability and rehabilitation ; 6)
1. Handicapped - Employment 2. Vocational rehabilitation
331.5'9

ISBN 1-85302-235-7

Printed and Bound in Great Britain by
Athenæum Press, Gateshead, Tyne and Wear

Contents

Introduction: Vocational Rehabilitation and 1992 *Michael Floyd*		1

Part I: A United Kingdom Perspective

1. A Follow-Up Study of Accident Victims 13
   Paul Cornes
2. Training and Enterprise Councils and the Economic and Social Renewal of Britain 22
   Frank Coffield
3. Vocational Rehabilitation Services in the United Kingdom 37
   Michael Floyd
4. Supported Employment in Great Britain 43
   Adam Pozner
5. What should a Good Vocational Rehabilitation Service provide? 52
   Katherine Floyd

Part II: A European Perspective

6. Maastricht and Vocational Rehabilitation 59
   Donal McAnaney
7. Lessons form the First Horizon Programme 76
   Erwin Seyfried
8. The Helios Programme 83
   Elizabeth Chennell

Part III: An American Perspective

9. Vocational Rehabilitation Research in the United States of America 91
   Fred Menz

Contributors 132

Introduction
Vocational Rehabilitation and 1992

Michael Floyd

This book was originally going to be simply a collection of papers presented at a conference, on 'Vocational Rehabilitation and 1992', which the Rehabilitation Resource Centre organised in March, 1992. However, due to delays in getting final versions of some of the papers and the consequent dating of some of them, I have asked some of the authors to revise their papers so as to make them more relevant to the current vocational rehabilitation scene. I have also requested additional contributions which cover topics that were not dealt with at the conference due to the unavailability of central government speakers – due to the impending election – and of speakers from the European Commission – partly due to a hiatus in the Helios programme.

What we have now, though, in this final collection of papers is, I think, a really excellent overview of the challenges facing vocational rehabilitation services in the United Kingdom and of the ways in which our membership of the European Union can help us to meet these challenges.

Furthermore, represented amongst the contributors to this book are a number of people who I believe have made a major contribution to vocational rehabilitation practice in Europe and the United States. Their thinking, some of which is very clearly outlined in these papers, will hopefully have a very significant influence on future policies and practices in the UK and in Europe.

Changes in the Labour Market

The need for new thinking, and for a more radical review of current approaches to vocational rehabilitation, has become extremely urgent as a result of major changes in the labour market. It is just over 20 years since an unemployment level in excess of a million was greeted with horror and dismay. Now we are invited to hail a decline to levels in excess of two million as an important achievement by the government. And there are many who would argue that the real level is much higher, well in excess of three million.

It is generally recognised too that disabled people are disproportionately represented in both the group of all unemployed people and, more importantly, those that have been out of work for more than a year. A survey of disabled people in the workforce (Prescott-Clarke 1990) estimated that just over one million people in the workforce could register as disabled and that, of those, over two hundred thousand were unemployed.

It is also likely that many of the approximately one and a half million disabled people, who are in receipt of invalidity benefit, would be capable of employment, if it were available. Another survey, this time of all disabled people (Martin, White and Meltzer 1989) found that there were approximately two million disabled people of working age (16–25) and that only 31 per cent of them were in employment.

Unfortunately neither of these 'one-off' surveys make it possible to identify what the long-term trends are but there is certainly a concern that disabled people are actually being affected more by these changes in the labour market, in spite of the various vocational rehabilitation programmes and government policies, such as the Quota Scheme, designed to ameliorate their situation.

We should also bear in mind that these changes may be affecting particular groups of disabled people more than others. Thus, for example, people with psychiatric disabilities are almost certainly experiencing even higher levels of unemployment than those cited above. And young disabled people, like young people from ethnic minorities, are probably experiencing very high levels of unemployment. Recently it has been estimated that over half of young, black people in Britain are unemployed. Hopefully the figure for all young disabled people is not quite so bad but it is not likely to be much better.

These changes pose a number of major dilemmas for vocational rehabilitation (VR):

- should open employment continue to be the primary goal for those using VR services?
- are the changes that have taken place in the labour market over the last 30 or so years likely to continue, so that the opportunities for entering open employment are going to deteriorate even further?
- if open employment is no longer a primary goal, or if it becomes an increasingly unattainable one, what should it be?

The Impact of New Technology

For some time now most commentators have tended to attribute the changes, that have taken place in the labour market, to the impact of new technology. There has been surprisingly little examination of its impact on disabled people in particular, but those that have addressed this issue have inclined towards an optimistic view.

Thus at an Anglo-German conference I helped to organise ten years ago, looking at the impact of new information technology, most of the contributors emphasised the positive aspects:

- New information technology, it was argued, would make it possible to reduce, or even eliminate, the handicapping effect of many disabilities
- It might also make it possible to make changes to the organisation of many jobs so that disabled people would be able to do them

- In particular, it would be possible for disabled people to tele-work, i.e. work from home using a computer terminal, so that the physical inaccessibility of many work-sites would no longer be a problem.

Only two of the conference papers addressed the more difficult issue of how new information technology might affect the labour market, both in terms of the number of jobs and in terms of the types of jobs. Considerations of this kind result in a less optimistic view. Thus, over the last few years, there has been increasing evidence (see, for example, McRae 1994) that new technology is having a major impact on the numbers of unskilled jobs. In the developed world at least, the number of these jobs has declined very significantly and is likely to go on declining.

There is a growing awareness that these changes are having a devastating effect on certain groups of people, and on society as a whole. A recent article, in *The Guardian* newspaper, suggested that, in the US, young black Americans had been particularly affected by these changes and that this was, in turn, responsible for the amazing statistic that indicates that one-third of all black Americans are either in prison or on parole. There is no evidence that disabled people in the US have been affected to quite this extent. There is however a concern that many disabled people in the UK used to find employment most readily in unskilled employment and that many of these openings no longer exist. Prejudice has undoubtedly played a major part in forcing many disabled people into less skilled jobs than they are capable of doing. None the less there is also evidence (Prescott-Clarke 1990) that many disabled people do not have the skills that developed economies increasingly require, and that this is due to the barriers they face in accessing appropriate education and training.

Other Changes in the Labour Market

While there is a growing recognition of the significance of these changes and their implications for the even greater priority that needs to be given to vocational training, there are a number of other changes in the labour market that receive less attention and yet call for equally radical changes in vocational rehabilitation services.

Foremost amongst these is the decline in jobs in the manufacturing sector and the growth of the services sector. In another Anglo-German conference paper, Whitehead (1985) was drawing attention to this phenomenon and the need for sheltered workshops to adapt to these changes. Since then a switch from manufacturing to services has proceeded apace, and has been especially marked in the UK and the US economy (McRae 1994). The chapter presented by Frank Coffield explores some of the issues raised by these changes.

Another very significant change, which is also receiving increasing attention, is the increased insecurity which very large sections of the working population are experiencing, with fewer and fewer people able to contemplate a 'job for life'. The occupational stress associated with these changes is almost certainly going to increase the numbers of those experiencing psychiatric disabilities, but they will also present new challenges to other groups of disabled people. Some writers, such as Handy (1995), foresee radical changes in the way in which individuals and employing organisations relate to each other and, in particular, a tremendous growth in the numbers of self-employed people.

As with new technology, several writers have welcomed this growth and see it as a liberating force as far as disabled people are concerned. The reality may however be less attractive and amount to little more than an increase in insecurity and home-working, as far as most disabled people are concerned. Research carried out by Frank Coffield and his colleagues also points to the problems associated with well-meaning attempts to help disabled people by means of so-called 'enterprise training'.

There has been surprisingly little discussion of how VR services need to change in order to meet the very different needs of disabled people in the twenty-first century. One notable exception was a very thoughtful and perceptive monograph, which Paul Cornes, another contributor to the conference, prepared over ten years ago for the World Rehabilitation Fund.

The monograph (Cornes 1984) outlines some very interesting and original ideas that have been developed in a number of other countries, regarding the choices that society will have to make in relation to these issues. These choices will not only affect disabled people but also many other disadvantaged groups, including those already mentioned such as young people and people from ethnic minorities. One possible scenario is that such disadvantaged groups become increasingly marginalised, becoming part of what some have termed an 'underclass'. Cornes points out that the effects of this could be lessened if attempts are made to ensure that even those who are excluded from participating in the economy receive a proper income enabling them to enjoy a reasonable standard of living.

Or, it can be argued, society can attempt to intervene in the labour market so that the level of unemployment does not rise any further, more jobs are created and paid work is shared out as equitably as possible. The European Commission White Paper on employment argued strongly that such a policy was not only possible but that it was highly desirable. The UK's Conservative government has however inclined to the view that governments can – or should – only exercise very limited influence over the economy. These tensions found their most obvious manifestation in the debates over the Maastricht Treaty and, in particular, in the 'opt-out' exercised by the UK in relation to the Social Chapter. A fascinating and insightful account of how the Maastricht Treaty may affect disabled people is provided by Donal McAnaney's chapter. He also discusses further changes that are needed in European policy, if the employment prospects of disabled people are to improve, instead of deteriorating further.

Policy Options

If we are to develop more appropriate and more effective policies that will ensure that, in spite of these challenges, disabled people will at least 'hold their own' in the labour market, if not improve their situation, then we must also examine very carefully the policy options that are available.

One of the most important benefits that may result from a study of policies and practices in other countries is that it can make us aware of alternative ways of tackling difficult problems. This is certainly the case with regard to social welfare policies and, in particular, with policies relating to disability and employment. I have argued, on a number of occasions, that the UK can learn much from Germany (Floyd and North 1991). Experience there has demonstrated, for example, that a Quota Scheme can work and that, given the right legislative structure, most employers will comply. Other aspects of the German system – the protection against dismissal given to disabled employees, the statutory right to representation of disabled employees, the very impressive vocational training provided for workers who become disabled – all warrant very close examination for the lessons we can learn from them.

Much can be learnt from other countries as well. One of the most comprehensive comparisons of policies in other countries was recently commissioned by the Department of Employment. In the report of the study (Lunt and Thornton 1993) policies and services in 15 different countries are examined. The authors have subsequently published a very interesting monograph (Lunt and Thornton 1995), in which they develop an interesting framework, within which these different approaches can be analysed and compared in a more systematic way. They identify four different types of measure that can be used to improve the employment circumstances of disabled people:

- policies of obligation, such as quota schemes
- policies that emphasise individual responsibility by protecting or promoting 'the position of disabled people seeking, or in, employment', e.g. protection against dismissal
- policies of persuasion, where the emphasis is more on persuading employers of the advantages of employing disabled people and on providing financial assistance, such as with technical aids and adaptations, and incentives such as those provided under the job-introduction scheme and the Sheltered Placement Scheme
- policies, whose aims are to make the individual more competitive, such as those governing the provision of vocational rehabilitation and training services.

In a fascinating comparison of rehabilitation approaches in the US and in the UK Stubbins drew attention to the excessive emphasis, in the US, that was placed on this fourth area of policy (Stubbins 1982) He suggested that, although vocational rehabilitation services in the UK were much less professional, and perhaps therefore less effective, the UK system did not neglect totally the importance of other measures.

His argument could be rephrased, using Lunt and Thornton's terminology, by saying that in the UK more emphasis was placed on policies of obligation, such as the quota scheme, and on policies of persuasion. It could even be argued that the UK has been, for much of the last 50 years, world leader in this respect. Any claims to such leadership today have however been undermined by the government's failure to enforce the Quota Scheme. Furthermore, the adoption in the US of the Americans with Disabilities Act (ADA) has meant that the US, which has for some time had much more professional and sophisticated vocational rehabilitation services, can now claim to also have the most advanced policies of 'obligation'.

I was therefore especially pleased when Fred Menz agreed to come over and present a paper at the 'Vocational Rehabilitation and 1992' conference. His chapter provides some fascinating insights into how much we can learn from the US.

Anti-Discrimination Legislation and Beyond

At the time of the 'VR and 1992' conference, the likelihood of anti-discrimination legislation being adopted in the UK did not appear very great. Since then however a very effective campaign has been fought, with groups of disabled people very much in the vanguard, to get such legislation through the British Houses of Parliament. Aided by sympathetic Labour MPs, such as Alf Morris and Roger Berry, and with the expert assistance of disability organisations, such as RADAR (Royal Association for Disability and Rehabilitation), legislation similar to the ADA has nearly reached the statute book. The Conservative government has however just managed to block it on each occasion, but has been compelled to bring in its own Disability Bill. Although much weaker, and less comprehensive than the ADA this Bill none the less represents very substantial progress. Together with the new Code of Practice for employers, it will have a very significant impact on employment opportunities for disabled people. And hopefully before too long a Labour government will introduce measures, such as a Disability Commission, which will greatly enhance its effectiveness.

There is a danger though that this major achievement, with regard to policies of 'obligation', will divert attention and effort away from other equally important areas. Groups of disabled people have been especially inclined to concentrate all their attention on this one aspect of policy, arguing that the 'social model' of disability implies that attempts to help the individual are misplaced.

The need for further progress, in the three other areas of policy, is however as great as ever, if not greater because of the labour market changes outlined earlier. One area, in particular, holds out tremendous promise. Supported employment is an approach that was developed in the US during the 1980s and has now become one of the most exciting and promising type of provision in Europe. An Association of Supported Employment Agencies has been formed (Ogilvie 1995) as well as a transnational, European one. Adam Pozner's chapter, based on research carried out since the 'VR and 1992' conference, provides a very useful overview of how this whole area is developing.

There are some, who would argue that, given appropriate and well-resourced supports, most disabled people could be employed in ordinary work situations. In other words, there will eventually be no need for sheltered workshops. British government policy does in fact envisage a gradual shift of sheltered employment away from workshops towards sheltered placement schemes. There is a need though for caution here. Relatively few people with psychiatric disabilities have been found sheltered placements. This could be simply because insufficient resources have been made available by the Department of Employment. Given the full range of support individuals need, it may well be that most could function in a sheltered work setting.

But, as the research reported by Fred Menz makes clear, the level of resources needed may be very great indeed. As with community care, there may be a question mark over whether society is really prepared to make available the resources that are needed.

I think it likely therefore that there will continue to be a need for something like a sheltered workshop, though it may look very different from the ones around at the moment, such as those managed by Remploy. A much more appropriate model may well be the 'social firms', or 'social enterprises', that have been so successful in Germany and Italy. Only a few initiatives of this kind have been successful so far in the UK but hopefully we may see many more develop over the next few years.

Research and Development

I hope too that over the next ten years we shall also see the emergence, in the UK, of a significant and properly resourced research and development programme. Fred Menz's chapter provides a fascinating insight into the importance accorded to research in the US and by its federal government, in particular. It may be fanciful to suppose that the British government will ever set up a National Institute for Disability and Rehabilitation Research, with a budget of over $100 million a year. But perhaps we can begin to envisage something at the European level. A network of universities is already being established, hopefully with some support from the European Commission's research programme.

Such a network could build on the work described by Erwin Seyfried and Elizabeth Chennell in their chapters on the Horizon and Helios programmes. A number of possible research and development themes can be identified. For example:

- in-depth evaluative research, targeted particularly on new innovative projects, such as social enterprises, funded by the Horizon programme
- comparative studies of policies in different countries and of the outcomes achieved, including those relating to numbers of disabled people in work, unemployed etc.

One area in which I would particularly like to see a major R&D effort made is the introduction of modern approaches to management into rehabilitation centres and sheltered workshops. At City University we have begun to take some exploratory steps in this direction. These have been focused on the management philosophy and ideas of Edward Deming, whose work is believed by many to have provided the basis for Japan's remarkable economic achievements. Only in the last ten years or so have companies and other organisations in the West begun to apply his ideas. Up until now few rehabilitation organisations in the UK have done so but in the US some interesting attempts have been made and a useful report has been published by the National Rehabilitation Association (Mason and Stukie 1994).

Deming's ideas are, I think, especially interesting because one of his fundamental assumptions is that production 'failures', inefficiency etc. are seldom the fault of the individual worker, but are usually due to the 'system', i.e. those factors under the control of management. The poor productivity of disabled workers is usually assumed to be due to their disabilities, or lack of 'motivation', skills or whatever. The application of Deming's ideas would suggest looking instead at the management system in, say, a sheltered workshop.

Not only might application of these ideas improve the efficiency of workshops – and therefore, hopefully, the remuneration of disabled workers, – such workshops could become a much better 'advertisement' for disabled workers. What kind of message to prospective employers is provided by the amazing statistic that each employee in a Remploy workshop requires a subsidy, from the taxpayer, of over £7000 a year?

Improving the management skills of the staff of sheltered workshops and other rehabilitation centres is just part of the much broader educational programme that is needed to ensure that the services that are offered to disabled people are provided by properly trained, professional staff. Here again we in the UK lag a long way behind the US, which has over 100 Masters programmes in such areas as rehabilitation counselling, vocational evaluation, disability management etc.

To meet the needs, identified by the participants at the conference, and summarised in Kathleen Floyd's chapter, calls for a huge expansion of provision of this kind, as well as the development of National Vocational Qualifications at other levels, i.e. 2, 3 and 4. It also calls for the setting up of professional associations and of procedures of accreditation similar to those in the US. One of the very practical outcomes of the 'VR and 1992' conference has been the establishment over the last few years of the Vocational Rehabilitation Association.

Hopefully during the next few years we shall see the establishment of a European association of this kind. Meanwhile I hope that the following chapters will make it clear why we need such an association and will help to put some 'flesh on the bones' of the various ideas I have touched upon in this brief introduction.

References

Cornes, P. (1984) *The Future of Work for People with Disabilities: A View from Great Britain*. New York: World Rehabilitation Fund.

Floyd, M. and North, K. (1991) 'Disability and employment in Britain and Germany.' In M. Floyd and K. North. *People with Disabilities: Improving Civil Service Employment Opportunities in Britain and Germany*. London: Anglo–German Foundation.

Handy, C. (1995) *The Empty Raincoat*. London: Arrow.

Lunt, N. and Thornton, P. (1993) *Employment Policies for Disabled People* (ED Research Series No. 16) Sheffield: Employment Department.

Lunt, N. and Thornton, P. (1995) *Employment for Disabled People*. York: University of York Social Policy Research Unit.

Martin, J., White, A. and Meltzer, H. (1989) *OPCS Report 4: Disabled Adults: Services, Transport and Employment*. London: HMSO.

Mason, C. and Stukie, T. (1994) *Adopting TQM to Vocational Rehabilitation*. Boston: American Rehabilitation Association.

McRae, H. (1994) *The World in 2020*. London: Harper Collins.

Ogilvie, S. (1995) 'The association of supported employment agencies.' *ReHab NetWork*, Autumn.

Prescott-Clarke, P. (1990) *Employment and Handicap*. London: Social and Community Planning Research.

Stubbins, J. (1982) *The Clinical Attitude in Rehabilitation: A Cross-Cultured View*. New York: World Rehabilitation.

Whitehead, A. (1995) 'Recent developments in sheltered employment in Britain.' In M. Floyd and K. North *Disability and Employment in Britain and Germany*. London: Anglo–German Foundation.

PART 1

A United Kingdom Perspective

CHAPTER ONE

A Follow-Up Study of Accident Victims

Paul Cornes

Introduction

This topic can be addressed from different angles. One would be to adopt a social administrative framework to consider relevant legislation and policy over the years. Another would be descriptive, providing an account of vocational rehabilitation services now in place and how they have evolved. However, the former approach might be found to be too dry and academic and, given an inevitable reliance on official reports and publications as primary sources, the latter might be considered to provide an unwarranted endorsement of official policy and services, overlooking alternative ways of meeting needs. Neither approach would provide the consumers' perspective that is essential for a more widely ranging evaluation of the extent to which the needs of people with disabilities for assistance with vocational rehabilitation have been met in the past, or – looking ahead – what may need to be done to develop and provide more effective help in future. This presentation therefore adopts a third and, hopefully, more pragmatic approach, rooted in the experiences of people with disabilities and drawing on various outcomes from an extensive research programme conducted over the past decade by the Disability Management Research Group (DMRG) at the University of Edinburgh. Detailed reports on that research have been published elsewhere (references follow below). The aim here is to report some general findings which may serve to highlight shortcomings in current vocational rehabilitation policy and services and to illustrate the possible shape of more effective alternatives.

The Disability Management Research Group Programme

The DMRG programme was not focused on all people with disabilities but, rather, on accident victims. They were persons of working age who were injured at work or in road traffic accidents, whose injuries resulted in permanent disablement and/or an absence from work of at least six months, often much longer, who subsequently pursued compensation claims for their personal injuries and related losses. Subjects comprised a national sample including both men and women (with the former outnumbering the latter by a ratio of three to one) of all ages (fairly evenly spread from 16 to 65 years) and from all occupational skill levels (from unskilled manual workers to senior executives). The majority of their injuries were graded as 'moderately severe' or 'severe' on the Abbreviated Injury Scale, a standard clinical measure, with such injuries typified by long bone fractures involving joints in 'severe' cases (thus with the added risk of future osteoarthritis). However, there were also small subgroups of persons whose injuries were classified as either 'minor', for example, mechanical injuries of lumbar or cervical spine not involving the spinal cord, or 'serious', such as traumatic amputations, spinal cord injury resulting in paraplegia or tetraplegia or head trauma resulting in brain injury. [For further information, see Cornes, Bochel and Aitken (1986); Cornes (1992)].

Before the DMRG programme was undertaken, there were no published data on clinical, social and occupational characteristics of accident victims. Provision of such information therefore was a primary objective. Another main aim was to record the nature and extent of the involvement of those persons with various British services which provide assistance with rehabilitation and return to work. That aspect of research yielded clear evidence of a disparity between timescales for medical treatment and settlement of claims. Whereas, on average, definitive medical treatment was concluded in less than one year, most claims took, on average, around three years to settle. The two-year lag between medical and administrative timescales directed attention to what happened during that interval.

Further scrutiny of the data indicated that a majority (around two-thirds) of the accident victims returned to work before settlement of their claims. That finding was in strong contrast with previous literature on compensation claimants, which has had an undoubted emphasis on 'compensationitis', 'compensation neurosis', 'secondary gain', 'malingering', 'exaggeration of symptoms' and other similar reactions to pursuit of a compensation claim, and which has given a clear impression that such reactions were commonplace. That widely-held impression was not supported by DMRG data, which found that evidence or suspicions of such responses to involvement in litigation were restricted to fewer than one in ten cases. The DMRG results therefore support the conclusions of Weighill (1983), who reviewed previous literature on compensation neurosis and concluded that previous studies had presented a biased picture based on non-representative sampling procedures.

Nevertheless, whilst a comparatively high proportion of personal injury claimants returned to work on completion of medical treatment and before settlement of their claims, a substantial minority who were medically fit to resume employment did not do so. Those were persons who potentially should have benefited from referral to vocational rehabilitation services, including occupational therapy and Department of Employment specialist services for people with disabilities. But further review of data indicated that fewer than one in 20 personal injury claimants had been referred to those services for advice or assistance. Given that occupational therapy services are rarely available to UK hospital orthopaedic department out-patients, where the majority of accident victims received follow-up treatment following relatively brief in-patient stays, infrequent referrals to that profession may not be surprising. It may be considered more surprising that so few accident victims were referred, or referred themselves, to Department of Employment services. It is understood that, with the latter Department, there is a circular instruction advising staff against involvement in cases in which there are unsettled personal injury claims. If so, the reasons for that instruction may require elucidation and, if necessary, wider debate amongst all concerned.

Factors Associated with Return to Work

Having examined personal injury claimants' characteristics and their involvement with rehabilitation and resettlement services, the DMRG programme turned attention to factors associated with return to work. That interest was triggered in part by analysis which showed that four-fifths of all accident victims who returned to work before settlement of their claims did so within a year of injury and which indicated that clinical variables – on which much medical advice on fitness for work is based – are not clearly linked to vocational outcomes. Systematic testing of the latter hypothesis entailed two studies. The first was a detailed content analysis of medical reports prepared for medicolegal purposes (Cornes and Aitken 1992). The second comprised a literature review of variables thought to be predictive of vocational outcome as a preliminary to more detailed analysis comparing accident victims who returned to work with those who did not using both univariate and multivariate statistical procedures (Cornes 1988). The latter study both confirmed that clinical variables were poor 'predictors' of vocational outcome and yielded an alternative, mainly non-clinical prediction model which discriminated between returners and non-returners to work with 94 per cent accuracy.

The indication that outcome at settlement was 'predictable' stimulated interest in a new problem. Was it possible to identify, amongst persons who have not returned to work within a year of injury, those who might be helped to do so by referral to appropriate services? If so, could that be done using information that was routinely available or which could be obtained during that time? Statistical analysis revealed that there were seven items of information which distinguished persons who returned to work within a year of injury from those who did so later or not at all. Those variables were age, gender, occupational skill level, length of treatment, local labour market conditions, presence or absence of a spinal injury and presence or absence of psychological problems of adjustment. Simply (i.e. nominally) scaled in accordance with the percentage of persons in each scoring category who returned to work, those seven variables were combined to form the Vocational Rehabilitation Index (Cornes 1990; Cornes and Roy 1991). A claimant's VRI score is the sum of his or her ratings on all seven items, and will fall somewhere between the minimum of 7 and the maximum of 24, with higher Index scores indicating greater levels of need for referral for help with vocational rehabilitation.

Detailed review of individual case histories and further statistical comparisons between persons whose scores fell into each of four VRI score bands suggested another application. The Index could also be used as a guide to the kind of help needed by, and the most appropriate vocational objectives for, persons whose scores fell into each band (Cornes 1990).

Lower range VRI scores (7 to 11) were recorded for 30 per cent of personal injury claimants. Generally, this group included higher than average proportions of males, younger people, persons employed in professional/managerial or skilled manual occupations, and persons whose injuries were classified as severe. No psychological problems were recorded for this group and four members with whiplash injuries were not deterred from resuming employment soon after injury. Because 86 per cent returned to work within a year of injury and 97 per cent did so before settlement, members of this group had minimal needs for referral to vocational rehabilitation, although some late returners might have benefited from relevant information or advice.

Lower middle range scores (12 to 14) were recorded for 33 per cent of the sample. Members of this group included higher than average proportions of younger people, persons employed in professional/managerial, skilled manual and semi-skilled manual occupations, and persons whose injuries were classified as severe. They also included about two-thirds of all persons noted to have experienced post-traumatic neurosis (normally treated successfully by family doctors) and around two-thirds of all persons with comparatively minor injuries to the neck or spine. Less than half (45 per cent) returned to work within a year of injury and only two-thirds (68 per cent) had done so by settlement. Individual case histories suggested that many non-returners might have benefited from early counselling and advice, involving their employers wherever possible, with a view to retention in their pre-accident occupations. Alternatively, the aim would have been another full-time job in the open labour market.

Upper middle range scores (15 to 17) were recorded for 26 per cent of sample members. This group included higher than average proportions of females, older people, persons in lower level 'white collar' and semi-skilled manual occupations, and persons with moderately severe injuries. They also included around one half of all persons with comparatively severe psychological problems and a similar proportion of all claimants with low back pain, although one half of the whole group suffered from neither condition. Also many members of the group had resigned or had had their employment terminated in the period after injury. Only 10 per cent of this mainly middle-aged, poorly-skilled and unemployed group had returned to work within a year of injury, rising to 24 per cent who had done so by settlement. Some of its members' needs for rehabilitative assistance could have been met by counselling and advice, but mostly their needs were much greater – for occupational assessment, followed by employment rehabilitation or training in a new occupation. In almost every case, though, the ultimate objective should also have been full-time, competitive employment in the open labour market.

Upper range scores (18 to 24) were recorded by the remaining 11 per cent. Members of this group comprised two main categories. The first included mainly elderly persons who had suffered apparently minor injuries of the lumbar spine (male unskilled manual workers) or the neck (females in professional or managerial occupations), with histories of chronic pain and, in some cases, suspected functional overlay. The second included younger persons who had suffered serious injury, frequently involving damage to the brain or spinal cord, resulting in very severe residual physical and psychological disabilities which rendered them unfit for employment on the open market. Only 5 per cent of this group managed to return to work before settlement of their compensation claims. Case studies suggested that it was quite unlikely that the needs of this group could have been met by conventional vocational rehabilitation services. Some might have benefited from specialised programmes dealing with chronic pain or the psychological problems they experienced. But, even if such interventions worked, it was doubtful whether persons in this group would have succeeded in the open labour market. Part-time or supported employment, placement in a sheltered workshop or, for the most severely disabled, diversionary occupation in a day centre for the physically handicapped would have been more realistic objectives for such persons.

Development of techniques to assist the early identification of potential non-returners or late returners is only a partial solution. There is much evidence to suggest that conventional management of disability practices do not put patients in touch with rehabilitation services at the earliest, most opportune time and that there is a requirement for better co-ordination in the delivery of needed services. That evidence led to thinking about a new question. Given that so many accident victims had so little contact with the existing services, was it possible to develop and implement services to improve the return-to-work rates for those people? Further consideration of this problem provided an opportunity to consider the nature of services that would be required to meet more effectively the vocational rehabilitation needs of not only accident victims but also other people with disabilities. A main theme of such thinking was the requirement for a professionally-oriented service, ideas which were first mooted over a decade earlier in reports from the Employment Rehabilitation Research Centre (Cornes 1982 et al.), but which seemed to have been buried in the darkest cupboards of the Department of Employment.

A Case Management Service

A first chance to explore and evaluate alternative professionally-based services arose in liaison with a private-sector insurance company. That company, NEL Britannia (now UNUM plc) was helped to train nurses who were employed to provide a counselling and case-management service to its permanent health insurance claimants (Cornes 1986). That innovative service seems to have thrived and expanded, and it is believed that the company has plans to develop it still further. The service was modelled on an approach that will be very familiar across the Atlantic and elsewhere in the world – a case-management approach, based on careful assessment and the development and implementation of a rehabilitation plan linking clients to relevant services.

Initially, it was considered that the main requirement was for a co-ordinating role of that kind. Indeed, it was on that basis that the DMRG launched a similar service for personal injury claimants within the framework of a random allocation controlled trial (believed to be the first of its kind in vocational rehabilitation in the UK), in which clients were allocated either to an experimental group in which they received the new service or to a control group in which they were left to find their own way for six months before switching over to receive the service on a deferred basis (Davey, Cornes and Aitken 1992). At this point in time, it is not possible to provide detailed results. However, it is possible to share some preliminary findings.

First, there was evidence that, even in apparently straightforward cases (of, for example, lower limb fractures), patients do have difficulties in getting back to work, but they can be helped by this kind of service. It is possible, therefore, that a large number of patients currently reviewed in Orthopaedic out-patient departments without careful consideration of need for assistance with vocational rehabilitation and referral to relevant services could be helped by such provision.

Second, there was an indication that positive outcomes, in terms of getting people into vocational training and/or employment, were more likely to occur in the second six months of service delivery. In other words, in the region of one year's sustained casework was needed to achieve resettlement. That, of course, holds very clear implications regarding the need for help of a very different kind from that which has typically been provided through our Jobcentre-based Disability Employment Adviser service.

Third, there did not seem to be any indication from control group members who were left to their own devices for six months, that they pursued vocational rehabilitation on their own initiative, for example, by contacting Disability Employment Advisers and/or other Department of Employment specialist services for people with disabilities. Existing services, therefore, were not providing them with an effective bridge to return to work. Rather, it was discovered that much more than a co-ordinator's role was called for, and that the co-ordinating function needed to be backed by a range of other assessment, case management, counselling, problem-solving and job development skills of the kind for which Rehabilitation Counsellors in other countries are prepared in the course of their extensive professional training.

From a more general perspective, in planning and conducting its research programme, the DMRG read and heard quite a lot about financial disincentives to pursuit of vocational rehabilitation. Not surprisingly, that topic is very prominent in discussions of compensation claims. But DMRG evidence does not suggest that it is always a major problem. Indeed, as noted above, the majority of people whose cases were studied returned to work before their claim was settled. Also, pursuit of a compensation claim did not undermine commitment to the random allocation controlled trial. Nevertheless, financial disincentives cannot be overlooked and there are problems in this area which still need to be addressed, including the interrelationship between incapacity and unemployment benefits and the need for a partial disability benefit.

Another issue concerns the effectiveness of Department of Employment specialist services for people with disabilities. Today it is very difficult to evaluate such services because official statistics focus on throughput (the number of persons in contact with services) rather than placement effectiveness (the number who actually get jobs). DMRG results highlighted just how few potentially eligible clients have any contact with specialist services and the very small number who were thereby helped into employment.

DMRG work also underlined the complexity of the system, most graphically demonstrated by Blaxter (1976). Her mapping of services within one Scottish city clearly illustrated how many different agencies, organisations and professions are in some way involved in the field of rehabilitation. It must be doubtful if any participant in that complex network could draw accurately those parts of the map which do not refer directly to their own services. Yet it is expected that individual people with disabilities should be able to find their way round that maze unaided. The pressing need for a co-ordinating function could not be more clearly illustrated – although, as previously indicated, co-ordination needs to be reinforced by other professional services.

Regrettably, better co-ordination has proved very difficult to achieve because generally British policy and services have been developed from a sequential model of disability management. That traditional model assumes that medical, social and vocational aspects should be dealt with in turn as an individual 'progresses' through different stages of recovery. Consequently, any employment problems are the last to be tackled, sometimes – if not often – years after injury or impairment. In contrast, other countries clearly recognise the requirements for concurrent management of all of those aspects. Britain also requires services to bridge all of these medical, social and occupational dimensions. Without bridging there are delays and the longer the delays, the less likely it is that clients will get back to work. Early intervention is critical and all rehabilitation policy and practice should be clearly guided by that principle.

Looking to the Future

In Britain, such principles have proved virtually impossible to apply in practice because of the fragmented nature of service provision. That, in turn, can be traced back to the original blueprint for policy and services drawn up over 50 years ago by the Tomlinson Committee. The deliberations of that Committee took place during the Second World War and in the context of more widely ranging concern over wartime labour market requirements. They also took place against a backdrop of pre-war debate on such topics as workmen's compensation, the training and resettlement needs of disabled ex-servicemen and the rehabilitation of persons injured by accidents which had found very little consensus between the various parties involved. The medical profession pressed to oversee an expansion of medical rehabilitation which would incorporate vocational services. Trades unionists were keen to preserve hard-won entitlements to financial compensation and were prepared to concede a role for rehabilitation only in relation to their own members, because they feared that an extension to non-members would render them fit to compete for their members' jobs. Government, chiefly through the (then) Ministry of Labour, was strongly opposed to the introduction of professional rehabilitation services of any kind.

The outcome was that the Disabled Persons (Employment) Act 1944 (which put the Tomlinson Committee's recommendations into effect and which has cast a long shadow over virtually all subsequent provision to help people with disabilities enter or return to work after illness or injury) was, and has remained, essentially a bureaucratic solution imposed top-down and based on minimal labour market research or consultation with relevant professions and clients or consumers. Small wonder, therefore, that the organisation, scope and effectiveness of Tomlinson-inspired services have been subject to mounting criticism or that various official reviews – often resulting in changes of name (or acronym) rather than function – have not yielded significant changes in philosophy, policy, practice or effectiveness. The quota scheme remains toothless and unenforceable. Advice and assistance to the vast majority of jobseekers with disabilities is still regarded as an executive rather than a professional task. Help continues to be deferred until involvement with medical and other services has ceased. And the Ability Development Centres (the rump of Employment Rehabilitation Centres) continue to operate with a staffing structure that was developed not for people with disabilities but for the Civilian Resettlement Units set up during the Second World War to assist the psychosocial readjustment of former members of the armed forces.

In the half century since Tomlinson, there have been radical changes in the labour market, both nationally and internationally. A post-industrial economy demands post-industrial vocational rehabilitation policies and practices. Further tinkering with the Tomlinson inheritance therefore should be regarded as no longer acceptable. More radical change is needed if people with disabilities are to achieve a fair share of employment opportunities in the years ahead.

Future developments should be considered in a much wider context and should also reflect the changing aspirations and empowerment of people with disabilities, although such changes are as yet more evident in other countries than in Britain. However, even this country, it is unlikely that the door to anti-discrimination legislation will remain permanently shut. Legislation of that kind should pave the way for two developments. One would be a shift of focus from provision of services, including assessment services, regardless of their relevance to client need. The other, reflecting decisions already made in such other countries as Canada, Australia and New Zealand (all of which have tried and rejected the British approach), would be the implementation of new professional services. These would be rooted in both public and private sectors and based on widely-ranging evaluation of the kind of service needed both now and in future. The DMRG's research and development programme might be considered to exemplify some aspects of service provision that will be needed in future.

Taken into account alongside developments in other countries – particularly those which have tried but now abandoned the British approach – it is difficult to avoid the conclusion that today's successful interventions by Department of Employment specialist services for people with disabilities are achieved despite rather than because of the quintessentially bureaucratic system in which they are obliged to work. Almost certainly, if British vocational rehabilitation policy and services had been based on the bottom-up, client-focused, needs-based approach now so widely adopted by other countries, it is quite improbable that we would be obliged to face the future with the pattern of provision we have today.

References

Blaxter, M. (1976) *The Meaning of Disability*. London: Heinemann.

Cornes, P. (1982) *Employment Rehabilitation: The Aims and Achievements of a Service for Disabled People*. London: HMSO.

Cornes, P. (1986) 'At last a rehabilitation counselling service.' *Post Magazine and Insurance Monitor 147*, 32, 22–23.

Cornes, P. (1988) 'Predicting return to work after injury.' *Journal of Rehabilitation Sciences 1*, 138–141.

Cornes, P. (1990) 'The Vocational Rehabilitation Index: A guide to accident victims' requirements for return to work assistance.' *International Disability Studies 12*, 32–36.

Cornes, P. (1992) 'Return to work of road traffic accident victims claiming compensation for personal injury.' *Injury 23*, 256–260.

Cornes, P. and Aitken, R.C.B. (1992) 'Medical reports on persons claiming compensation for personal injury.' *Journal of the Royal Society of Medicine 85*, 329–333.

Cornes, P., Bochel, H.M. and Aitken, R.C.B. (1986) 'Rehabilitation and return to work of employer's liability claimants.' *International Journal of Rehabilitation Research 9*, 119–128.

Cornes, P. and Roy, C.W. (1991) 'Vocational Rehabilitation Index assessment of rehabilitation medicine service patients.' *International Disability Studies 13*, 5–9.

Davey, C., Cornes, P. and Aitken, R.C.B. (1992) 'Evaluation of a rehabilitation co-ordinator service for personal injury claimants.' *International Journal of Rehabilitation Research 16*, 49–53.

Weighill, V.E. (1983) 'Compensation neurosis: a review of the literature.' *Journal of Psychosomatic Research 27*, 97–104.

CHAPTER TWO

Training and Enterprise Councils and the Economic and Social Renewal of Britain

Frank Coffield

Introduction

Karl Popper in his intellectual autobiography *Unended Quest* (1976, p.124) argues that the only excuse for giving a lecture (or writing a paper) is to challenge the audience. I shall try to live up to that advice in this chapter by using the evidence presented by Michael Porter (1990) in his book *The Competitive Advantage of Nations*, where he studied the exporting record of ten major countries, including Japan, West Germany, Italy, the United States and Britain. His first conclusion is that we must abandon the notion of a 'competitive nation' because no nation can be competitive in everything and instead we must focus on specific industries and particularly on geographic clusters of similar industries, and, rather than looking at the total monetary value of the exports of leading firms, he examined their share of world markets. In effect, he set out to answer this central question: how do firms in particular countries achieve international success in distinct industries?

His conclusions make grim reading for a British audience. His figures, for instance, show that Germany continues to have a broad industrial and manufacturing base, with its leading firms in chemistry, mechanical engineering and physics sustaining their international advantage by moving into more and more sophisticated areas. When we turn to Japanese firms, their top ten exports accounted for from 82 per cent to 59 per cent of world markets in these areas: motor cycles, TV recorders, dictating machines, calculating machines, mounted optical elements, photo apparatus, cameras, cash registers, piston engines and electric gramophones. Clearly, Japanese firms have invested heavily in the advanced new industries, which utilise high technologies and high skills and, as a result, have come to hold a commanding share of world exports in these commodities, while failing in many others such as chemicals. We have witnessed in the last 20 years a major shift in economic power to Japan, and it is Michael Porter's thesis that we shall see in the next 20 years more economic power moving to Japan and to other Pacific countries like Korea and Singapore because their leading companies relentlessly upgrade their competitive advantage by continual innovation.

Japan's economic success since 1945 has been the focus of much discussion in the West, but less so the Italian economy. It is not widely known in this country that Italy recorded the second highest rate of growth anywhere in the world (and second only to Japan) since the Second World War, but it is highly unlikely that this comparative success can be attributed to the Italian education and training systems. Porter's analysis of both Italy and Japan makes clear that there is no simple or direct connection between investment in education and training and superior economic performance, as both countries are struggling to modernise their educational systems. His sophisticated model of competitive advantage should at least make us question the assumption, which is widely prevalent in Britain today, that our economic decline can be traced back solely or principally to deficiencies in our systems of vocational education and training.

Porter entitles the section on this country 'The Slide of Britain' and emphasises how our industrial performance is a 'mixture of both success and failure, a point easily lost in focusing on the problem areas' (p.482). But compare the top ten UK industries in terms of their share of world exports with the Japanese list given earlier: whisky, aircraft, aircraft engines, cast iron scrap, antiques, diamonds, hand paintings, wool, high carbon steel and cinema film. These industries accounted for 78 per cent to 25 per cent of world markets in these commodities and is obviously a more varied list than that of Japan. He concludes that Britain will not regain its competitive advantage over other countries '...without a world-class educational and training system encompassing all socioeconomic and ability levels'. For Porter, a first-class educational and training system, open to all sections of the community, is a necessary but not a sufficient condition of international success. There are many other determinants of national advantage but this is not the place to discuss them further and readers are referred to the model described in his third chapter (p.69ff.). Porter's figures, arguments and conclusions are only part of a growing body of evidence (e.g. Wiener 1981) which details the economic decline of the UK and which has consequences for us all. The rest of this chapter will examine some of the strategies for economic and social regeneration which have been introduced by Conservative governments since 1979.

The Enterprise Culture

One of the catalysts for change chosen by Ministers has been a series of measure (see Coffield 1990) designed to move individuals and communities from 'the dependency culture' to 'the enterprise culture'. Adequate definitions of the two terms are hard to come by but Peter Morgan, Director General of the Institute of Directors, has supplied the following:

> An enterprise culture is one in which every individual understands that the world does not owe him or her a living, and so we act together accordingly, all working for the success of UK PLC...successful companies, which regularly make profit and grow, are the flagships of the enterprise culture. Directors who lead those successful companies are heroes of the enterprise culture... In an enterprise culture the whole nation understands that we are

locked in competition with other nations. We are all soldiers in a global economic war... (Morgan 1990)

Later in the same speech he identified three obstacles to progress: establishment attitudes, the middle-class salariat and the lumpen proletariat and then continued:

> What do I mean by our third obstacle, the lumpen proletariat? I mean the mass of the population we choose not to educate... Less educated people are less able to profit from the enterprise culture. Because they cannot profit from enterprise, they are thrown into the dependency culture... Our task is to deliver the goods – create the wealth – and win more hearts and minds for capitalism and enterprise... The government must keep the faith (Morgan 1990).

In contrast to the military metaphors and the rhetoric of the revivalist preacher, I would like to present the results of a small-scale piece of empirical research which my colleague, Rob MacDonald and I (MacDonald and Coffield 1991) completed in the county of Cleveland in North East England, which sought to evaluate the experiences of young entrepreneurs, participating in the Enterprise Allowance Scheme (EAS).

In more detail, we looked at the following groups: the self-employed (50); those who set up co-operatives (12); the previously self-employed, our euphemism for 'gone bust', (15); those previously in co-operatives (9); those in community enterprise projects, a particular form of non-profit-making enterprise (9); and 16 long-term unemployed people – 8 men and 8 women of the same age as members of a control group. In total we interviewed a sample of 104 including 5 from the ethnic minority community in Teesside, which is roughly their percentage in the local population.

The detailed analysis of the interviews suggested that our sample fell into three broad categories. First, 10 per cent proved to be successful in their new business ventures which is obviously of importance to them, their families and the locality; second, 20 per cent failed in their business or co-operative, some of them ending up with considerable debts (in one case of over £20,000); many more became physically and psychologically dejected. They reported to us that they had been told during their training on Enterprise Awareness Days how to set up in business but not when and how to cut their losses and how to wind up a failing firm.

The most surprising finding, however, was the largest of the three groups in the middle, the 70 per cent of 'plodders' (their term), who continued to work long hours for very low rates of pay. They had long since given up hopes of being successful and were struggling (and often failing) to achieve more modest ambitions – of making enough to live on. Their attempt at self-employment is more accurately described as a form of self-exploitation (Rainbird 1991).

One of the problems with the EAS is that each new cohort of enthusiastic entrepreneurs has to contend with earlier cohorts who were launched into self-employment by the same scheme; they draw up a business plan, examine the pricing structure of their competitors and then undercut their rivals to secure a corner of the market for their services. And virtually all our interviewees were in the service sector – mobile hairdressers, car valets, musicians, or picture framers. Storey and Strange's (1993) study of all new business in Cleveland during the 1980s showed that 26 per cent were concentrated in only two sectors: hairdressing or car-related activities. These findings expose the gap between the rhetoric of government on enterprise and the reality of local provision: does anyone seriously believe that the economy of Cleveland or of the North East will be regenerated by a growth in the number of beauticians, window-cleaners or cut-price, back-street car mechanics?

Certainly, our interviewees themselves entertained no such hopes for this government initiative. Although professing a general lack of interest in, or knowledge, of politics, they nevertheless understood that the main political objective of EAS was the 'register effect', namely, keeping their names off the unemployment register.

The Rise in the Peripheral Work-Force and Unemployment

There are also structural changes at work in the labour market which I wish to draw attention to. Catherine Hakim (1987) has pointed to the long-term growth in the size of the peripheral work-force, which she argues is made up of part-time workers and temporary workers as well as the self-employed. Looking specifically at part-timers, in 1951, 800,000 people worked part-time, which was only 4 per cent of the total work-force. By 1987, however, this number had increased to 5,600,000, or 23 per cent of the work-force. When government ministers talk about the huge rise in the number of jobs created in the 1980s, it is mainly part-time jobs that they are referring to.

This long-term trend has ushered in a new age of insecurity, where multinational firms export jobs to developing countries, slim down their 'core' work-force and subcontract services like maintenance, security and catering to smaller firms which often re-employ some of the same workers but at lower rates of pay and with inferior conditions of employment. The result is a growing army of casual, flexible workers on short-term and/or part-time contracts. Large public sector employers in health and education have increasingly followed the lead given by industry and commerce; they have responded to declining resources from central government by adopting the same strategy of engaging large numbers of part-time workers, mainly women, who have no hope of full-time, permanent contracts. In this way, sections of the British middle class are learning about the exploitation of staff with insecure or temporary jobs. Moreover, the experiences of working-class, redundant steel or ship workers in precarious, casualised labour markets are more reminiscent of working conditions in the nineteenth century than of a new era of enlightened management of human resources. To use the jargon, many employer practices seem more pre-Fordist than post-Fordist.

David Piachaud (1992) has similarly plotted the steady growth in unemployment over the same period of time, by calculating the average number of people unemployed in the UK in each of the last four decades:

1950s	338,000
1960s	459,000
1970s	976,000
1980s	2,714,000

Even more worrying is the rise in long-term unemployment, i.e. those out of work for over a year. In the early 1960s, the total stood at around 50,000 and today it is over one million (Employment Policy Institute 1993). Such long-term trends suggest that, even if the current recession were to end soon, it is highly unlikely that we shall ever return to the very low levels of unemployment (1 or 2 per cent) which characterised Britain in the 1950s and 1960s.

Training and Enterprise Councils (TECs)

The establishment of the TECs has been described by a former Secretary of State for Employment as 'one of the most radical and important initiatives ever undertaken in this country' (Gillian Shephard 1992). Again, the TECs have been chosen as a catalyst for change, both individual and corporate, by means of which the British economy is to break into new markets through massive investment in human capital.

We examined the progress made, and the problems faced, by the five TECs in the North East as a means of raising a number of key issues confronting the whole TEC movement. The conclusions are based on a series of interviews with TEC board chairmen and senior staff, with senior civil servants and upon an assessment of official documents and relevant literature.

Because the North East was one of the first regions to have all its five TECs up and running, it provided an ideal testing ground for independent researchers not only to chart progress so far, but to question whether the TECs, as presently constituted, are ever likely to fulfil the central remit laid down for them by government – 'to foster economic growth and contribute to the regeneration of the community they serve' (Department of Employment 1991, p.101). The rest of this chapter will present seven themes considered essential to the ability of the TECs to achieve this objective:

(a) Public accountability versus local freedom
The establishment of the TECs has resulted in a substantial redistribution of power and public resources from the Training Agency and local authorities to unelected groups of employers, who still argue that the new dispensation does not give them enough freedom if they are to achieve genuine and lasting change. Yet it is difficult to imagine any government of whatever political complexion giving more autonomy to 82 independent private companies (as the TECs are) to exercise in 82 different ways in 82 separate localities. The public debate has been largely concerned with the struggle between the TECs and the government over levels of funding and over the failure of some TECs, mainly in the south of England but not in the North East, to meet the guarantee of a training place to all school-leavers. There have been tensions at a deeper level. The government,

for its part, has been concerned to make the TECs publicly accountable, both nationally and locally; the TECs, on their side, have argued for greater freedom to respond to government priorities in ways that best suit local conditions.

TEC leaders have waged a semi-public campaign (with tactical leaks to the press) about the repeated cuts in their budgets and their wish to be involved in the formulation of policy. They also argue for the flexibility to switch resources from one heading to another, to adapt national programmes (for example, Employment Training or Youth Training) to local needs.

Judith Marquand (1992, p.33) points out that, compared with the limited discretion of their predecessors, the Area Manpower Boards, 'TECs wield genuine power' and 'are building their power bases locally and collectively'. Currently, the TECs are pressing for funding based on performance and outcomes rather than on inputs and process (such as the number of training weeks). The Department of Employment, on the other hand, is concerned about the variable performance of the TECs, and has begun to develop a series of performance indicators.

What is less well developed is the accountability of the TECs to their local communities. The annual reports produced by the North Eastern TECs more closely resemble promotional material than statistical accounts of the previous year's performance. Achievements in YT or ET (and particularly the rates of job placement and qualifications gained) could be recorded in regional and national league tables in the same way as the attainments of school pupils are being made available to parents and the general public, provided the proper allowance is made for levels of attainment on entry to such courses. The annual publication of comparative statistics on training those with special needs, a constituency which has so far been seriously neglected by the TECs, would most effectively demonstrate the TECs commitment to the entire communities they serve. Without such publically available data, it is impossible to judge the performance of the TECs. Interestingly, in July 1993, David Hunt, the Secretary of State for Employment, announced that TEC 'league tables' would be published in order to stimulate higher levels of achievement.

The outcome of this struggle will be fascinating to watch because leading industrialists have the ear of the present government in a way that trade union leaders have not, as the abolition of the National Economic Development Council in June 1992 demonstrated. If employers, acting in concert and privately threatening to resign in droves, cannot wrest more independence and resources from this government, then no one can.

(b) What role?
When appearing before the employment committee of the House of Commons in June 1991, Roger Dawe, director general of the Training, Enterprise and Education Directorate (TEED) of the Department of Employment, claimed that 'the *raison d'être* of the whole TEC movement is the training of the employed'. Yet one of the most recent publications of the Department of Employment (1993, p.4) points out that YT and ET account for 86 per cent of TEC expenditure. This is a central contradiction at the heart of the TEC initiative.

The tension over the TECs' role, then, is whether they should be managing social programmes for underprivileged groups or stimulating local economic development. The extra responsibilities which have been heaped upon the TECs since their inception (examples from the 1992 Budget include Learning and Training for Work, Work Start and TEC Challenge), have not helped the development of a coherent strategy. In the words of Michael Hanson, chief executive of South Thames TEC, they have been involved in an 'alphabet soup of initiatives' (1992, p.51).

The government has also failed to develop a regional strategy for the TECs. In November 1991, the Secretary of State for Employment issued guidance to the TECs on developing the national framework but only 'at national, sectoral and local level' (Dept of Employment 1991, p.10). The need for a regional dimension is perhaps more obviously seen by the nine TECs which have been created to serve London. Labour markets do not neatly coincide with TEC boundaries and so for some initiatives a regional approach is necessary. At present, the five TECs in the North East meet to discuss boundary disputes and the agenda of G10 meetings. But policy on issues like inward investment, tourism, high technology, relationships with higher education and the European Single Market needs to be developed on a regional basis.

The regional offices of TEED could be given the strategic role of involving all interested parties in developing, implementing and evaluating a regional development plan. The prospects, however, of the present government devolving policy, finance and implementation to locally accountable bodies in the regions are almost nil; and yet, as Irene Brunskill (1990, p.5) has contended, if 'local economic development [is not] firmly set within a national and EC policy framework [it] is doomed to failure'. Regions such as Catalonia in Spain or Bayern in Germany have set up offices in Brussels to lobby hard for increased aid, but the Northern region was at first represented solely by Wearside TEC. Although this development shows considerable innovative drive, it has to be asked whether it makes sense for all 82 TECs in England and Wales and the 22 LECs (Local Enterprise Companies) in Scotland to open offices in Brussels. In effect, all five TECs in the North East have since combined to make common use of the Brussels office and so some acknowledgement has been made of the fact that the rest of Europe is organised regionally.

(c) Change: voluntary or legislative?
In the white paper *Education and Training for the 21st Century* (Major 1991, p.38), the government stresses that the commitment of employers to training is to be secured by voluntary means 'without the damaging consequences of compulsion.' The bureaucratic burdens of the previous levy system are advanced by government and some employers as reasons for rejecting regulation. These are genuine difficulties but the case *for* legislation still deserves to be heard.

First, a growing body of evidence points to the widespread and hazardous failures of the present market in training, of which the best-known example is the 'poaching' of trained workers by companies not prepared to invest in training. Group training schemes and centres would help to eliminate 'poaching' and, if properly inspected and assessed, would ensure a minimum standard of training throughout industry and commerce as part of a national system of certification.

Second, the onus is on the proponents of voluntarism to state how long it will take for the policy to work. How many years will it be before most firms in the UK have been awarded the insignia of Investors in People (IiP), an initiative to encourage world-class standards in training and staff development? According to the regional director of TEED, 16 firms from a total of 218 employing 200 or more people in the North East became IiPs in the first six months of the scheme up to the end of May 1992, and a further four in the subsequent year to May 1993. The national figures (Mills 1993) reveal that, out of approximately 5000 companies employing 200 or more people, only 288 had achieved the status of IiP by June 1993.

Officials in four out of the five TECs studied said that personally they did not foresee voluntarism working and favoured some form of legislation. Exhortation, leading by example and insisting on contract compliance on issues of quality may not be enough to change the anti-training culture of most medium and small companies in Britain. Codes of good practice and gentle persuasion have not led firms with 20 or more workers to employ a quota (currently 3 per cent of the work-force) of registered disabled people. The quota scheme was introduced in 1946 and 41 years later in 1987 'only a quarter were in line with or above the required percentage' (Morrell 1990, p.1). It is not an offence for an employer to be under quota. If Britain has to wait 40 years to involve 25 per cent of employers in training, we shall be witnessing the most protracted revolution in recorded history.

Third, as Peter McBride (1990 p.76) has rightly argued, 'the former levy system had the great merit of placing the financial burden where it belonged, i.e. on the industries which would benefit'. No enlightened company would be in the least threatened by, and would have much to gain from, a law which, for example, required 1 or 2 per cent of total payroll to be spent on employee training by those firms which do not train to national standards.

Finally, legislation would neither break new ground nor involve the abandonment of any principle because the government has had recourse to law to enforce change in education. Besides, the construction industry and the construction sector of the engineering industry already operate a statutory levy system and 'an overwhelming majority of members within both sectors favour [its] continuation' (CBI 1989, p.38). In sum, the arguments for legislation are powerful; they have convinced both the German and French governments.

(d) Market forces versus strategic planning

When arguing for the establishment of the TECs, the CBI (ibid., p.37) stipulated the central mechanism to be introduced: 'a market should be created to allow individuals and employers to exercise choice and to influence the nature of vocational education and training on offer locally.' This exhortation had, of course, direct appeal for a government whose central policy since 1979 could be described as setting Britain free from state intervention, planning controls and over-regulation.

What advantages have so far accompanied the setting up of a free market in training? The TECs, as regulators of the new training market, now have the power to weed out the providers of poor quality training by imposing rigorous control. The North Eastern TECs claimed that they were now much more selective about what courses ran, and were able to specify the level and type of training required by local employers. Some of the colleges of further education have, however, complained that instead of an open system of bidding where all providers compete on equal terms, the local TEC has awarded contracts directly to the private sector and has been unwilling to discuss this apparent bias.

Moreover, the government aim of improving the choice of individuals in training is often irrelevant because, as Phil Hodkinson (1991, p.83) has pointed out, 'employers not students are the clients of FE. Therefore, if employers want training in a limited range of job-specific skills, that is what they are given'. In what is supposed to be a free competitive market, one set of employers applies to another on the Board of the local TEC for public funds to run training courses tied to the completion of National Vocational Qualifications (NVQs), which are based on competences assessed in the work-place by the first set of employers.

The experience of YTS further suggests that 'without intervention, markets cause employers to *avoid* costly training' (Lee *et al.* 1990, p.185; emphasis in original). The funding arrangements for TECs will encourage them to train those who are likely to achieve NVQs in the shortest possible time and to neglect those with special training needs or those aiming for high level skills which would be costly to provide. The Department of Employment (1991, p.12) had to intervene in the workings of the market by awarding in 1990–91 £12 million of 'bonus awards' to those TECs which exceeded training targets set for the proportion of people with disabilities, or from the ethnic communities, or from the long-term unemployed.

Market forces also tend to encourage short-term decision making rather than long-term strategic planning; and historically in Britain training budgets have been cut at the first hint of a recession. The 'short-termism' of British industry is being matched by the 'short-termism' of government's treatment of the TECs. Although TECs must produce a three-year corporate plan, funding from the Treasury is allocated on a yearly basis which creates uncertainty, inefficiency and the fragmentation of policy. The evaluation by David Lee and his colleagues of YTS in a prosperous South Eastern town led them to the conclusion that:

> The government is going in precisely the wrong direction in equating the behaviour of individual employers with the public good. It is useless in a system whose whole rationale is based on short-term competitive individualism to expect hard-pressed employers to behave altruistically with an eye to the long-term public interest...individual employers will only invest in workers they intend to use for their own production needs. (Lee *et al.* 1990, pp.192–3)

Above all, this debate has become absurdly polarised between those who criticise 'exclusive reliance on market forces', on one side, and those who oppose 'bureaucratic state control', on the other. Since the steep rise in youth unemployment in the mid 1970s and the urban disturbances of the early 1980s, governments of both main political parties have intervened on an unprecedented scale in the training market with an avalanche of measures aimed at young people and adults alike. The issue at stake, however, is not whether to intervene in a free market, but whether the interventions that have been made form a coherent strategy likely to succeed.

(e) Training: generic versus customised
The last few years have witnessed the development of a remarkable consensus over the need for a national framework for training, a consensus which has been supported by the CBI (1989), the Trades Union Congress (1989) and the All Party Select Committee of the House of Lords on the European Communities (1990). The CBI then produced *World Class Targets* (1991) in education and training which have received very wide and deserved support. There is a danger that the huge mobilisation of effort needed to move towards these targets will be considered sufficient on its own to transform Britain's industrial performance. Such arguments have become, in Tony Cutler's (1992, p.180) provocative words, 'politically convenient...because they fit so neatly into a model where the less affluent regions must pull themselves up by their bootstraps'. They also divert attention away from other, more radical measures such as investing in British manufacturing industry or devolving power to the regions or developing a national, industrial strategy. The chief executive of Cumbria TEC in his letter to the Employment Committee of the House of Commons summed up the point: 'the local problem is greater than a mismatch of skills to vacancies, but one of a dire absence of jobs of any sort.'

The letters from TECs to the Employment Committee also provide evidence of how Employment Training has come to be regarded as 'providing customised training to exactly meet employers' needs'. Such narrow, job-specific training is in stark contrast to that currently provided by major employers in Germany, where, for instance, the company AEG (1991, p.4) stresses the need for both practical and theoretical knowledge: 'the new professions...require the training not only of technical job content but in addition [the development] of personal and social skills [which] lead to an overall professional competence.' In Britain TECs appear to be more concerned with quantity than quality; and training is so illiberally conceived by some employers that employees may constantly need to be retrained rather than given an understanding of change and how to cope with it.

When the rate of entry into jobs after ET (30 per cent nationally), and the number of trainees gaining qualifications (again 30 per cent) are considered, the continuation of the whole programme is brought into question. The problems with YT are similar; in 1990 41 per cent of trainees gained a qualification, but that proportion had dropped to 31 per cent by 1993 (*Labour Market Quarterly Report* 1993, p.8). What educational course would be allowed to continue with failure rates as high as these?

(f) Enterprise
Alongside the two ugly sisters of ET and YT, enterprise has remained Cinderella, who still awaits the transformation that will sweep her off to the ball. In the

strategic guidance issued to TECs by the Secretary of State for Employment in both 1990 and 1991, the encouragement of enterprise was the sixth and last priority for action. In 1990–91, expenditure on business enterprise support amounted to only 3.5 per cent of total TEC expenditure (Department of Employment 1991, p.12).

All five North Eastern TECs have set up a network of customer support services and have appointed a director for enterprise and economic development. Although all five claimed to have become more selective in supporting new ideas through a revamped Enterprise Allowance Scheme, the contribution of self-employment to the economic regeneration of the region is likely to remain important but limited for reasons given earlier.

In some of the TECs we heard of a culture clash between a proper concern for following well-tried administrative procedures on the part of cautious civil servants and the desire for new, quick and flexible action by thrusting entrepreneurs on the board. Nationally, the rhetoric of government continues to stress the creation of an enterprise culture, but the political will to fund enterprise support programmes appropriately is missing. The enterprise movement remains a bandwagon in search of definition.

(g) Business Education Partnerships
Business Education Partnerships are meant to bring coherence and quality to a range of initiatives undertaken by the two sectors. Britain, however, remains a seriously under-educated and untrained society. Whatever the past failings of individuals, institutions, governments and employers, the National Education and Training Targets (NETTs) now set out eight clear objectives (see *Employment Gazette* July 1992, p.344) by which to measure progress from our relatively low starting-point.

These targets provide the opportunity to leave behind the unhelpful dialogue of the 1980s between business and education. All the relevant parties now need to come together in a strategic alliance to work jointly towards the achievement of these targets. The national and local partnerships between business and education will be tested to the full, with the targets providing a hard edge by making both sides accountable for change and monitoring their performance.

The TECs have been given a leadership role in the attainment of the national targets and they have been urged to structure their business plans around them. Such measurable objectives should help focus activity in an area which has so far been characterised by a plethora of well-meaning, but poorly co-ordinated, initiatives. The TECs, however, will not be the only organisations put to the test. The education and training systems must now be galvanised into action and into greater co-operation than ever before.

Four criticisms deserve, however, to be made of the NETTs. First, compared with the equivalent targets set by countries such as France, Korea or Thailand, they constitute a poverty of expectations and a minimal level of achievement. Second, as with all reform in education and training in recent, the targets have been imposed from above without consultation with those who now have the responsibility of reaching them. Third, the prime movers behind the targets were not government ministers (who had to be dragged into line), but the CBI and senior civil servants in the Department of Employment. The group whose support is conspicuous by its absence is the Department for Education and Education Ministers. Indeed, the latter responded to the rising numbers of sixteen-year-olds passing GCSE examinations in 1992 by claiming that standards in education were being diluted rather than rising. Finally, as Ewart Keep (1993, p.3) has pointed out, there remains a more fundamental problem still with NETTs, namely, 'a lack of demand within the British economy for the levels of skill which the targets specify'.

Conclusion

This chapter began by assessing the challenge to Britain's future as seen by Michael Porter, a professor from the Harvard Business School, and has then continued by evaluating some of the key government strategies for economic and social regeneration. The subsequent sections on the enterprise culture, the structural changes to employment and unemployment, and the establishment of the TECs prompt the conclusion that two government strategies are being employed simultaneously.

The first rhetoric of government argues that the UK must produce a more highly educated and trained workforce to ensure that British companies compete successfully in high technology markets, where advanced skills, flexible specialisation, and sophisticated management techniques result in full order books, high wages, and continual innovation. The NETTs are the outward, visible manifestation of this strategy which could be summarised as follows: long-term investment – high skills – high productivity – high wages and successful competition based on quality.

At one and the same time, government action – such as the abolition of the Wages Councils which set statutory minimum hourly rates of pay for 2.6 million low-paid workers, opposition to the Social Chapter and a minimum wage, legislation which has created the most deregulated labour market in Europe – suggests that a second strategy is being vigorously pursued. Competitive advantage is also being sought at the bottom end of the market. Hence the advertisements placed in German newspapers in June 1993 by the Department of Employment advertising the low wage rates obtainable in the UK. This approach could be characterised as: short-term investment – low skills – low wages – and successful competition based on low costs.

Instead of seeing these two policies as mutually incompatible and contradictory, it may make more sense to interpret them as part of one coherent plan for different sections of the community; the former for the future managers, professionals, scientists, technologists and senior administrators and the latter for the growing army of part-time and peripheral workers, the under-employed and the unemployed. Although John Major in the Foreword to the white paper *Education and Training for the 21st Century* (1991) claims that the government 'will end the artificial divide between academic and vocational qualifications', the *actions* of successive Conservative governments have served to widen that gap. For example, the A level examination, the traditional but heavily criticised (DES 1988) route to higher education, has been defended and shielded from much-needed reform, while new curricula (e.g. BTEC courses), offering low-level, 'transferable' skills in a wide range of occupations, have been promoted for millions of flexible, casual workers.edThe announcement by Education Secretary, John Patten, in July 1993 that in future the General National Vocational Qualifications (GNVQ) at Level 3 or Advanced Level will be known as the 'vocational A level', now creates three separate pathways for the 16–18 age group. First, the academic route through A levels – 'traditional A levels remain a cornerstone of our policies' (Patten 1993) – remains sacrosanct and unreformed. Second, the new GNVQs will provide a vocational route for those in full-time education and are aimed at 25 per cent of the age group. And finally, NVQs will offer a vocational route for those who leave school at 16. Although the attempt to raise the prestige of vocational qualifications is to be applauded, the Government have recreated a socially divisive, tripartite system post-16 which will not win parity of esteem for the three pathways. Instead we need a more radical measure of the kind Michael Porter advocates which would introduce one unified qualification system at 18, where students from all types of background could take a combination of academic and vocational modules.

The danger in pursuing these divisive strategies simultaneously is that the social polarisation, which researchers like Pahl (1984) have pointed to, is likely to be intensified and legitimated. Instead of seeking greater social cohesion, social justice and social solidarity with the unemployed or those with special training needs, the creation of markets in education and training is steadily widening the divisions between the haves and the have-nots.

To arrest our economic decline, I could envisage a government gaining widespread support for unpopular long-term measures (such as increasing the standard rate of taxation to pay for increased investment in education and training) by arguing that 'we are all in this together' and that 'sacrifices, commensurate with ability to pay, will have to be made by all sections of the community'. But what chance of success has a policy which, on the one hand, treats three million unemployed as the acceptable price of beating inflation, while, on the other, refusing to condemn the huge rises in directors' salaries which are unrelated to the performance of their companies (Gregg 1992)? The introduction, for instance, of both a minimum and a maximum income would signal a national determination to pull together towards the goal of economic and social regeneration. The fact that the first measure has been repeatedly rejected by this government and the second is nowhere discussed in polite company shows the extent of our social divisions. It also suggests, to me at least, that, in the absence of a more coherent and socially just programme for economic and social renewal, our economic decline is more likely to continue than to be reversed.

References

AEG (1991) *Training for the Future: The Integrated Training Concept.* Frankfurt/Main:AEG.

Brunskill, I. (1990) *The Regeneration Game.* London: Institute for Public Policy Research.

CBI (1989) *Towards a Skill Revolution.* London: CBI.

CBI (1991) *World Class Targets.* London: CBI.

Coffield, F. (1990) 'From the decade of the enterprise culture to the decade of the TECs.' *British Journal of Education and Work* 4, 1, 59–78.

Cutler, T. (1992) 'Vocational training and British economic performance: a further instalment of the "British labour problem"?' *Work, Employment and Society* 6, 2, 161–183.

Department of Education and Science (DES) (1988) *Advancing A Levels,* Higginson Report. London: HMSO.

Department of Employment (1991) *Training and Enterprise Councils and Vocational Training.* Memorandum to House of Commons Employment Committee. London: HMSO.

Department of Employment (1993) *TECs 1992.* Moorfoot, Sheffield: Dept of Employment.

Employment Gazette (1992) July.

Employment Policy Institute (1993) *Full Employment.* London: Employment Policy Institute.

Gregg, P. (1992) 'The disappearing relationship between directors' pay and company performance.' Unpublished LSE paper.

Hakim, C. (1987) 'Trends in the flexible work-force.' *Employment Gazette,* November, 549–560.

Hanson, M. (1992) 'TECs in London.' *Policy Studies* 13, 1, 46–53.

Hodkinson, P. (1991) 'Liberal education and the new vocationalism: a progressive partnership?' *Oxford Review of Education* 17, 1, 73–88.

Keep, E. (1993) 'National targets, training markets, and the demand for skills.' University of Huddersfield conference paper, July.

Labour Market Quarterly Report (1993) May.

Lee, D. et al. (1990) *Scheming for Youth – a Study of YTS in the Enterprise Culture.* Milton Keynes: Open University Press.

Major, J. Rt. Hon. (1991) 'Foreword.' *Education and Training for the 21st Century.* London: HMSO, CM 1536.

Marquand, J. (1992) 'Evaluation, decentralisation and accountability.' *Policy Studies* 13, 1, 30–39.

MacDonald, R. and Coffield, F. (1991) *Risky Business? Youth and the Enterprise Culture.* London: Falmer Press.

McBride, P. (1990) 'Towards a skills revolution: a summary and critique of the CBI report of 1989.' *The Vocational Aspect of Education* XLII, 112, 75–80.

Mills, L. (1993) 'Investing in people – a TUC perspective.' Speech at Conference, University of Huddersfield, 9 July.

Morgan, P. (1990) Address to the Institute of Directors Annual Convention, Royal Albert Hall, 27 February, 1–15.

Morrell, J. (1990) *The Employment of People with Disabilities: Research into the Policies and Practices of Employers.* London: Department of Employment, Research Paper No. 77.

Pahl, R.E. (1984) *Divisions of Labour.* Oxford: Basil Blackwell.

Patten, J. Rt. Hon. (1993) 'Patten announces vocational A levels.' *Department for Education News* 227/93, 8 July.

Popper, K. (1976) *Unended Quest*. London: Fontana.

Porter, M. (1990) *The Competitive Advantage of Nations*. London: Macmillan.

Rainbird, H. (1991) 'The self-employed: small entrepreneurs or disguised wage labourers?' In A. Pollert (ed) *Farewell to Flexibility?* Oxford: Blackwell.

Shephard, G. Rt. Hon. (1992) Speech to TEC Conference, 9 July, Metropole Hotel, Birmingham.

Storey, D.J. and Strange, A. (1993) *Entrepreneurship in Cleveland 1979–1989: A Study of the Effects of the Enterprise Culture*. Moorfoot, Sheffield: Department of Employment, Research Series No. 3.

Wiener, M.J. (1981) *English Culture and the Decline of the Industrial Spirit, 1850–1980*. Harmondsworth: Penguin.

CHAPTER THREE

Vocational Rehabilitation Services in the United Kingdom

Michael Floyd

The 1944 Disabled Persons Act

Vocational rehabilitation services were virtually non-existent in the UK prior to the Second World War. During the war, however, the government became increasingly aware of the need to provide such services if the large number of people injured in the war were to be able to return to employment. A committee, the Tomlinson Committee, was set up in 1941 and their recommendations were adopted in a very large measure in a major piece of legislation, the 1994 Disabled Persons Act (Bolderson 1991). This Act has shaped British vocational rehabilitation services during the last 50 years and no other legislation has been introduced during this period.

It offered four distinct means for helping disabled people:

- a Quota Scheme
- the establishment of Industrial Rehabilitation Units
- the provision of a resettlement (placement) service
- the setting up of sheltered workshops.

The Quota Scheme, like the quota schemes adopted in many other European countries, was very simple in concept. It stated that at least 3 per cent of the work-force of employing organisations should consist of registered disabled people. There were however important differences with regard to other such schemes, such as the West German one. Thus all central government organisations were exempt from the legislation. This was due to another significant feature: if organisations failed to comply with the legislation it was necessary to prosecute and then fine them. Over a period of 50 years only 11 such prosecutions have been made and the fines imposed have never been increased from the very low levels set in 1944 – just a few hundred pounds.

The Industrial Rehabilitation Units (IRUs) were established in most of the large cities and by the 1950s there were 27 of them. Each one offered a one-week assessment programme, followed by a rehabilitation programme which was spent in one of a number of workshops. Initially the IRUs were very successful and approximately three-quarters of the people using them were successful in finding employment.

The resettlement, or placement, services were provided by Disablement Resettlement Officers (DROs), who were based at the Ministry of Labour's local offices, which eventually became known as Jobcentres. The DROs helped individuals to find job vacancies and to apply for them. They referred clients to the IRUs and were responsible for determining whether individuals could be registered as disabled.

They were also responsible for judging whether they were likely to be incapable of working in open employment and should therefore be referred to a sheltered workshop. The government set up an organisation, Remploy, to run a large number of such workshops. Like the IRUs they were found in most cities. A few local authorities and large voluntary organisations also set up sheltered workshops and eventually around 15,000 disabled people came to be employed in them, each of them earning a proper wage, albeit a low one.

Developments in the Services, 1950–1980

Initially the Quota Scheme seems to have been quite successful and the level of compliance by employers was high. Gradually though the numbers of organisations achieving the 3 per cent quota declined and, in parallel with this, the numbers of disabled people registering as disabled also fell. The government came to believe, or at least to claim, that it was the failure of disabled people to register that meant that employers could not fulfil their quota. Organisations representing disabled people argued instead that it was the failure of the government to enforce the legislation that had resulted in there being no incentive for disabled people to register.

There was also a steady decline in the proportion of IRU clients going into employment. By the middle of the 1970s the proportion had dropped below one-half. A major evaluation of the IRUs, or Employment Rehabilitation Centres (ERCs), as they were called, was instituted. The report of the evaluation (which was one of the most thorough and comprehensive evaluations of a vocational rehabilitation service that has ever been carried out) was very critical of the ERCs. It pointed out that, apart from the change of name, there had been very few changes made in their rehabilitation programmes, in spite of major changes in both the kinds of disabilities their clients had and in the labour market. Their assessment techniques were also found to be very out-of-date (Cornes 1982).

There were however some more positive developments. Instead of concentrating all of the effort on changing and rehabilitating the individual, vocational rehabilitation services in the UK recognised that more needed to be done to tackle the barriers disabled people face in the employment situation itself. Thus, over the years a number of special schemes were introduced:

- help with fares to work
- providing advice, and financial assistance, with regard to technical aids that enable the disabled employee to carry out the job and with regard to adaptations to premises and equipment
- personal reader services for blind and partially sighted employees

- a small subsidy to employers for the first few weeks (job introduction scheme).

Developments During the 1980s

The very serious criticisms arising out of the evaluation of the ERC led to some fairly significant changes being made to the rehabilitation programmes being offered by the ERCs. The approach to assessment, in particular, was radically altered by the introduction of VALPAR work samples, imported from the US, and of more up-to-date psychometric assessments. New centres, known as ASSET centres, were also set up. These centres offered only assessment. Rehabilitation, which was provided in the artificial environment of a workshop in the ERC, was provided instead by local employers.

These changes represented however very limited progress. In the US a key resource for the vocational guidance and assessment services is an extensive database of occupational information, much of it available on computers. This makes it possible to match the functional abilities of the disabled client, as determined using the work samples and psychometric tests, to the mental and physical requirements of over 20,000 different jobs. In the absence of such information, relating to jobs in the UK, the new approach to assessment was inevitably 'half-baked'. Furthermore, in the ten years or so since the changes were brought in, no attempt has been made to address this problem.

Other changes though have had a more lasting impact. Perhaps the most successful of all has been the introduction of the Sheltered Placement Scheme. The 1944 Act had envisaged the possibility of small groups of more severely disabled people working in an ordinary employing organisation, but none the less being employed by another non-governmental organisation, which received a contribution from the government towards their wages, these being set at a level similar to that of the workshops.

This type of provision, sometimes referred to as enclaves or Sheltered Industrial Groups (SIGs), had not proved very successful, with only a few hundred sheltered employment places of this kind existing at the beginning of the 1980s. After much lobbying however the government agreed, in effect, to permit a SIG of just one disabled individual. This came to be known as a sheltered placement. The organisations employing the disabled person, the sponsoring organisation, pay them and receive from the host organisation, where the individual actually works, an agreed contribution towards their wage costs, proportionate to how productive they are assessed to be.

Another innovation, also reflecting the stronger orientation in the UK towards tackling the barriers disabled people face in the workplace, was the publication of a Code of Practice for employers (Manpower Services Commission 1983). This provided guidance to employers on a wide range of issues relating to disabled people.

The Code also provided a valuable reference for the Disability Advisory Service (DAS) teams that were set up at around the same time. These teams took over from the DROs the responsibility for working with employers, advising on technical aids, adaptations etc. and represented a further strengthening of the emphasis on overcoming barriers in the workplace. Considerable progress was also made towards the range and the amount of training provision that disabled people could access. The quality of this provision however continued to be very variable and to fall very far short of what was on offer in the West German rehabilitation centres.

More Recent Developments

In 1990 the Department of Employment published a major review of its services for disabled people (Department of Employment 1990). This review was, in part, a response to a fairly critical report produced by the government's National Audit Office (National Audit Office 1987).

Soon after the publication of the review, all the ERCs were closed and over 60 Placing, Assessment and Counselling Teams (PACTs) were set up, each serving a population of between half a million and a million people. The PACTs consisted mainly of DROs, now to be called Disability Employment Advisers, but also incorporated some of the staff from the ERCs, together with staff from DAS teams. Each PACT has around 15 staff, most of whom are based at Jobcentres (usually more than one).

Rehabilitation is now done by non-governmental agencies who are contracted, by the PACTs, to provide a rehabilitation programme similar in length to that offered previously by the ERCs. (For a more detailed account of the PACTs, see Williams 1993). Whether the service offered by PACTs is an improvement on that offered by the ERCs and ASSET centres remains to be seen.

The review also recommended a further shift, in sheltered employment provision, towards sheltered placements and away from sheltered workshops. At present there are still approximately 14,000 workshop places, but the number of sheltered placements has grown to around 6000, i.e. nearly a third of the total.

The most significant change during the last few years has undoubtedly been the introduction of anti-discrimination legislation. For several years now, the government has been blocking attempts, by individual Members of Parliament, to introduce legislation, similar to the Americans with Disabilities Act (ADA) which became law in the US in 1991. The pressure for such legislation, much of it coming from groups of disabled people themselves, had however become so great that the government was compelled to draft its own Disability Bill. This legislation is much weaker than the ADA, but none the less represents a substantial advance and it seems likely that a future Labour government will strengthen it further.

Looking to the Future

The changes I have described have very much the character of what we in Britain sometimes refer to as 'two steps forward, one step backwards'! Overall the vocational rehabilitation services for disabled people have probably improved, although this is not shown in statistics showing their participation in the labour force.

Thanks to higher levels of unemployment and other changes in the labour market, caused to a considerable extent by technological change, the numbers of disabled people seeking work is still very large, somewhere in the region of a quarter of a million. in addition to this 'visible' waste, there are a further one and a half million disabled people in receipt of 'invalidity' – or, as it is now to be termed 'incapacity' – benefit. Some of these are perhaps really incapable of work, at least in open employment, but it is likely that given really good rehabilitation, appropriate technical aids and adaptations and other forms of support in the work place, many of them could participate in the labour force. Hopefully the anti-discrimination legislation will help in this regard.

During the last few years though too much reliance has been placed on such legislation, especially by groups of disabled people. Organisations such as Royal Association for Disability and Rehabilitation (RADAR), have also tended to focus much of their afford in this area. I have argued elsewhere (Floyd 1995) that such legislation is essential but have pointed out that, as in the US, it needs to be backed up by really effective vocational rehabilitation services. And this means, in my view, developing more professional services, or, in other words, ensuring that the staff of rehabilitation centres have received proper training. (See also Cornes 1994.)

At present such training is almost non-existent. A very small number of Masters courses have recently been developed (Floyd and Smith 1994), including our own at City University. In the US however over a hundred such courses are offered. In the US there are also several professional bodies concerned with the accreditation of practitioners, such as rehabilitation counsellors and vocational evaluators. Hopefully something of this kind will develop over the next few years. In the UK we are setting up a Vocational Rehabilitation Association, but we should also be aiming, in the longer term, to establish a transnational, European body that could be the focus for accreditation of vocational rehabilitation professionals right across Europe or, at least, within the European Union.

References

Bolderson, H. (1991) *Social Security, Disability and Rehabilitation*. London: Jessica Kingsley Publishers.

Cornes, P. (1982) *Employment Rehabilitation: The Aims and Achievements of a Service for Disabled People*. London: HMSO.

Cornes, P. (1994) 'Challenges to development of effective disability management in the workplace.' *ReHab NetWork*, Winter.

Department of Employment (1990) *Employment and Training for People with Disabilities*. London: Department of Employment.

Floyd, M. (1995) 'Pre-employment screening and disabled people.' *Occupational Health Review*, May/June.

Manpower Services Commission (1983) *Code of Practice*. Sheffield: Manpower Services Commission.

National Audit Office (1987) *Department of Employment and Manpower Services Commission: Employment Assistance to Adults.* London: HMSO.

Williams, C. (1993) 'Life after the Consultative Document.' *ReHab NetWork*, Summer.

CHAPTER FOUR

Supported Employment in Great Britain

Adam Pozner

What is Supported Employment?

At the time of writing, there are approximately 120 Supported Employment agencies in Great Britain (National Development Team 1994). These agencies are currently supporting about 4000 people with disabilities into and within competitive open employment.

Although there are several usages of the term Supported Employment, the term is generally used in this country to describe the process of enabling a person with a disability to secure and maintain a paid job in a regular work environment, by supplying all appropriate training and support to them in the workplace where they will be doing the job (Pozner and Hammond 1993).

The following features are intrinsic to the Supported Employment model:

- Training and support are provided within the context of a real job and real workplace. The person is facilitated in developing the skills for the job they are going to do *in or around the workplace* where they will be doing it. It is a 'place and train (support)' as opposed to a 'train and place' model
- Job Coaches provide *all necessary support* that a person may need to do an identified job which may include training in job specific skills, help with travel to work, facilitating social interaction with work colleagues, or simply emotional and moral support. 'Natural supports' by workplace colleagues are developed wherever possible. Support is available on an *indefinite* basis and is often *intensive*, particularly in the early months of employment
- the model often involves specialist processes such as vocational profiling, job analysis, job development and systematic instruction. The latter offers a systematic framework for teaching job tasks broken down into simple key components to employees who have learning difficulties to meet their specific learning needs.

Supported Employment Versus 'Work Readiness'

Supported Employment challenges the efficacy of conventional work-readiness approaches where people develop transferable work skills within vocational training programmes or simulated work environments prior to employment.

Proponents of the Supported Employment model claim that work readiness approaches are ineffective for people with learning disabilities, as this group cannot easily learn and transfer generalised work skills from one job to another. Another criticism is that work readiness approaches often do not provide adequate workplace support to new employees and hence job retention is poor.

It is often said that people with learning disabilities have been failed by the whole emphasis on 'work readiness'. People 'prepare' for work indefinitely but rarely end up working. The low throughput from adult training centres, day centres and other work readiness programmes is often cited as a testimony to this failure.

Users

The vast majority of users of Supported Employment services in Great Britain are people with learning disabilities; however, a growing number of agencies are beginning to widen their clientele to include people with other disabilities, for example people with mental health problems and autism.

In the United States and within some European Union member states, Supported Employment services have been targeted to people with a range of other disabilities as well as learning disabilities. For example, approximately 15 per cent of agency users in the United States are people with mental health problems.

It is clear that current Supported Employment agencies in Great Britain are only reaching a small proportion of individuals who could benefit from their services.

The Department of Health has estimated that there are between 120,000 and 160,000 adults with severe or profound learning disabilities in England (Department of Health 1992). At 31 March 1991, there were 51,098 places in 620 adult training centres and 5625 places in 343 special needs units, a total of 56,700 places for people with learning disabilities in 663 centres in England (Department of Health 1991). Throughout from these facilities into paid employment has long been recognised to be minimal.

There is clearly unmet need among this population and several social service departments are working towards 'changeover' – the development of Supported Employment services rather than the diversionary day centre facilities. There is a growing trend among some agencies to work with younger people with learning disabilities of school age so that they never reach adult training centres.

Supported Employment and Mental Health

A growing number of agencies in Great Britain are beginning to deliver services to people with mental health problems who are also profoundly disadvantaged in the job market.

There are issues of programme design that must be carefully considered when developing services for this (and any) population. The types and patterns of support interventions required by people with mental health needs are likely to be different to those needed by individuals with learning disabilities. Rather than a focus on intensive job-specific skills training in the early months of employment, the emphasis is more likely to be on supporting an individual in coping with the work environment. Support may often be of an emotional or practical nature and may be required episodically over a long period of time, perhaps indefinitely. Those with intermittent or cyclical illness may require project-based employment opportunities or some system of absence coverage, which will allow them to have time off work without prejudicing their continued employment.

The Supported Employment approach will not, of course, be appropriate for all people with mental health problems. For those with higher support needs, other vocational service models may be more appropriate (social firms, clubhouses, transitional employment programmes).

Development of Supported Employment

Supported Employment agencies first made their appearance in North America and have expanded rapidly over the last ten years. Approximately 90,000 people with disabilities are being supported within employment by these agencies in the United States (Mank 1993).

Supported Employment is defined in the Developmental Disabilities Act of 1984, and in the regulations under the 1984 Amendments to the Education of the Handicapped Act and the Rehabilitation Act (Federal Register 1984). In the United States, it includes such models as enclaves, work crews, and entrepreneurial/workbench approaches, as well as individual placements within ordinary competitive employment. A criterion is also that working hours are at least 20 hours a week and clients are generally paid the market level wage rates.

There has been no single school of Supported Employment in the United States and there has been a range of approaches and viewpoints. Some of better known proponents are Bellamy (Bellamy, Horner and Inman 1979), Rusch (1986), and Gold (1975).

The economic viability and efficacy of the Supported Employment model as compared with more traditional service models has been examined through several longitudinal studies (Wehman et al. 1985; Schuster 1990).

It is claimed that such longitudinal studies have demonstrated the effectiveness of Supported Employment on every level including that of cost. This was made possible in the United States because of a Federal funding initiative and a benefits moratorium that provided the right conditions for Supported Employment projects to be able to prove their worth, without the constraining effects of the benefits system on client outcomes.

There are obvious valuable lessons to be learnt from the North American experience and readers are referred to the literature (Cioffi and Renes 1993; Pozner and Hammond 1993).

The Supported Employment model has taken root in a number of other European Union countries. Agency development is developing fast in the Republic of Ireland, Holland, Belgium, Portugal and Spain.

An embryonic European network, the European Association for Supported Employment, was established in 1993. The role of the the Association is to lobby at national and European level to ensure that future European programmes take account of the Supported Employment approach and dedicate resources to it.

In Great Britain, the development of Supported Employment has taken place more recently and on more modest scale. The first agencies emerged in the mid 1980s and growth has been sporadic. There are now somewhere in the region of 130 agencies in England, Wales and Scotland.

There is considerable ambiguity attached to the term Supported Employment in this country. The term has been adopted by the growing legion of specialist employment agencies providing workplace training and support, the subject of this chapter. However, the term is sometimes understandably used to refer to a wider range of sheltered employment models that provides a supportive work environment to disabled employees (e.g. sheltered workshops, enclaves, work crews and social businesses). Compounding this semantic confusion, the Employment Department has renamed its sheltered employment programme (workshops, factories and Sheltered Placement Scheme (SPS)) the Supported Employment Programme.

The Association of Supported Employment Agencies (ASEA) is an independent member organisation open to anyone interested in the development of Supported Employment in the United Kingdom. It was launched in 1991, following a conference aimed specifically at the needs of Supported Employment agencies. ASEA currently has something like 130 members. The Association has regional networks and special interest groups focusing on specific issues such as welfare benefits and marketing.

ASEA is concerned with establishing collective action on national issues that cannot be addressed by individual agencies. The Association is actively involved in liaison with central government, and in initiating joint national and European funding opportunities.

Its aims include the following: to endorse and promote quality standards in training support and development; to nurture and encourage the setting up of new Supported Employment services; to promote the training of the skills of Supported Employment throughout the UK and European Union; the provision of regular detailed information, advisory and development service to members and people with disabilities.

At the time of writing, the majority of Supported Employment agencies are funded by social service departments or health trusts. The sporadic distribution and development of agency provision primarily reflects local initiatives concerned with increasing throughput of day and residential service users into employment. Mainstream 'employment' monies have not been available until quite recently, although a few agencies have begun to tap into TEC (Training and Enterprise Council) and LEC (Local Enterprise Company) funding programmes (Training for Work, Local Initiative Funds, European Social Funds, TEC operating surpluses, National Development Programme) and Employment Department programmes (Agency Rehabilitation).

The Employment Department's Access to Work scheme which began operating in July 1994 may well be a significant new source of financial support for Supported Employment agencies and their clients in the future. The Scheme can fund a support worker if an individual needs practical support either at work or in getting to work. Each applicant will be eligible for financial support to the value of £21,000 over five years. However, at the time of writing there are still uncertainties over how eligibility criteria will be interpreted at local level, particularly with respect to those in receipt of incapacity benefits or therapeutic earnings.

The increased scope for funding through community care monies (Transitional Grant Monies and Care Management Budgets) administered by social service departments has also had an impact on Supported Employment provision. The requirement that 80 per cent of the former must be spent in the independent sector has provided an incentive for some agencies embedded in social service or health provision to move towards independent status.

Another important development may be the new funding framework underpinning the Employment Department's restructured Supported Employment Programme, which seeks to reward throughput from sheltered workshops and factories into employment. Just how this will impact on Supported Employment agency provision is uncertain.

National Development Team Survey

Research into Supported Employment in Great Britain is in its infancy; however, research initiatives are being developed at the universities of Durham, Birmingham, Cardiff and Kent.

The first national survey of Supported Employment in England, Wales and Scotland published by the National Development Team (Lister and Ellis 1992) provided us with our first broad overview of these agencies: the majority are set within social service day provision, but with a rapidly growing number of independent agencies; distribution is geographically sporadic with major clusters in Greater London, Wales, and the South East and North West of England; funding is piecemeal and fragile with little long-term funding; agency client profiles vary tremendously, but most agency clients are those with mild or severe rather than profound learning disabilities.

The survey revealed that agencies were succeeding in supporting their clients into paid employment, the majority securing part-time posts. The predominance of part-time employment reflects the impact of the benefits system rather than any deficits in working ability. Nevertheless, some 28 per cent of agency clients were earning more than £100 per week. 23 per cent of agency clients had stopped receiving any welfare benefits while 16 per cent had reduced the level of benefits received.

Job retention was excellent. While 14 per cent of agency clients leave employment each year only 4 per cent are actually dismissed from employment.

The survey showed clearly that employment is a real possibility for people with severe learning disabilities, many of whom have so often been labelled unemployable.

OUTSET Research 1993

In 1993 the Employment Department commissioned OUTSET's Consultancy Service to conduct qualitative research into Supported Employment. The aims of the research were to build up an up-to-date picture of Supported Employment in Great Britain, assess agency effectiveness and begin to identify components of good practice. The research was carried out by case-studies of ten agencies, a postal survey of TECs and LECs, consultation with key agencies working in the field, and documentary research (Pozner and Hammond 1993). The main findings of the research were as follows:

Efficacy

Agencies were *effective* in supporting large numbers of people with disabilities into ordinary paid employment, corroborating the findings of the National Development Team survey. Agency clients were finding real jobs with real wages in regular work settings. Posts were being secured in a wide range of occupational areas, primarily entry level posts within services industries. Job retention was excellent, agency clients maintaining posts for long periods of time.

Some agencies were able to support a higher proportion of their clients into full-time posts than others, though the reasons for this were uncertain. Many agencies reported few difficulties in finding suitable jobs for clients, even in areas of very high unemployment. There did not seem to be a correlation between agency outcomes and local unemployment levels, the major factor limiting outcomes was reported to be staffing limitations.

The benefits trap

Again, the impact of the benefits system on outcomes was clear. Many agency clients were restricted to part-time posts, not because they could not secure or retain full-time employment, but because they would be financially worse off or prejudice their housing situations if they worked longer hours. The impact of the benefits system remains the primary issue today for Supported Employment agencies.

Users

Many agencies were working successfully with people described as having severe learning disabilities, a group who historically have been labelled as unemployable, as well as with people with mild or moderate learning disabilities. Where agencies were including people with severe learning disabilities among their users, this was being achieved within reasonable programme costs.

It was also clear that the Supported Employment model can be utilised effectively within the framework of vocational training programmes. This approach enabled individuals with learning disabilities to sustain work experience placements and paid employment, who would not otherwise have been able to do so.

Good practice

Agency outcomes were reported to be enhanced by the following operational features: well-developed relationships with employers; a marketing approach that clearly emphasises programme benefits to employers; thorough vocational profiling, accurate job match and intensive workplace training; a powerful training technology; access to welfare benefits expertise; good liaison with Employment Service; and others. Further research is needed to examine more carefully the factors that make for effectiveness and quality outcomes in agency operation.

Costs and benefits

Costs associated with a client's intensive workplace training or support in the first year of employment may be significant, but are likely to decrease sharply thereafter. Subsequent 'maintenance' costs in future years are likely to be low for most clients with learning disabilities. The pattern may differ for clients with other disabilities and further research in this area is needed. Agency annual costs range widely between £1000 and £5000 per client supported into and within employment. The number of new clients supported into employment each year ranges between four and eight per agency job coach.

Agencies report improved quality of life, significant reductions in benefits take-up, and reduced usage of local day services after clients move into employment.

The study concluded that while there are indications of the long-term cost effectiveness of the Supported Employment model as an alternative to other more traditional approaches such as work preparation programmes and in reducing people's usage and dependency upon day services, longitudinal studies are needed to examine more rigorously the comparative efficacy of Supported Employment with other approaches.

In-depth cost-benefit analyses of Supported Employment agency operations are needed. These would allow clarification of the extent to which increased tax revenue and reduced benefits pay-out at Exchequer level might offset or even outweigh agency programme costs. They would also allow comparison of Supported Employment with other approaches, and identification of major cost factors.

Such analyses should take account of the quality of agency outcomes and social benefits, rather than simply adopting a purely financial model. It is also important that they be conducted over a sufficiently long time period for agencies to be able to demonstrate cost-effectiveness, that they take account of the effects of the benefits system on agency outcomes and of the contexts within which many agencies operate.

The Future

It is clear that the Supported Employment model has potential for many individuals currently disadvantaged in the labour market. It is likely that the next few years will see its application in many spheres. However it is important that future developments are informed by evaluation of existing programmes. It is also important that Supported Employment is seen as *one* option among many, a key feature of any local continuum of vocational opportunities.

References

Bellamy, G.T., Horner, R.H. and Inman, D.P. (1979) *Vocational Habilitation of Severely Retarded Adults, A Direct Service Technology.* Austin, Texas: Pro-ed.

Cioffi, A. and Renes, D. (1993) *Bibliography on Supported Employment*. Eugene, Oregon: University of Oregon, Employment Network.

Department of Health (1991) *Adult Training Centres for People with Learning Disabilities and Local Authority Day Centres for Adults at 31 March 1991 England, Personal Social Services – Local Authority Statistics*. London: HMSO.

Department of Health (1992) *Circular LAC (92) 15*. Department of Health.

Gold, M. (1975) 'Vocational training.' In *Mental Retardation and Development Disabilities: an Annual Review*, Vol. 7. New York: Brunner Mazel.

Lister and Ellis (1992) *Survey of Supported Employment Services in England, Wales and Scotland*. Manchester: National Development Team.

Mank, D. (1993) 'Supported employment in competitive work settings.' International Conference, June, Lisbon, Portugal. Unpublished.

National Development Team (1994) 'Work in the 21st Century for people with learning disabilities.' (Presentation at MENCAP conference in October, 1994)

Pozner, A. and Hammond (1993) *An Evaluation of Supported Employment Initiatives for Disabled People*. Employment Department, Research Series No. 17. Sheffield: Employment Department.

Rehabilitation Act Amendments 1986, [P.L. 99–506].

Rusch, F.R. (1986) *Competitive Employment, Issues and Strategies*. London: Paul H. Brookes.

Schuster, J.W. (1990) 'Sheltered workshops: financial and philosophical liabilities.' *Mental Retardation 28*, 4, 233–239.

Wehman *et al.* (1985) 'Competitive employment for persons with mental retardation: a follow-up six years later.' *Mental Retardation 23*, 6, 274–281.

CHAPTER FIVE

What Should a Good Vocational Rehabilitation Service Provide?

Katherine Floyd

Introduction

This chapter presents a summary of the discussions that took place in the first series of workshops at the conference. Participants were asked to imagine they had a variety of physical and sensory disabilities.

Workshop 1: Spina Bifida

Participants in this workshop were asked to consider what a good vocational rehabilitation service should provide, from the point of view of someone with spina bifida. They suggested that:

- the individual would want to have a realistic assessment of their own abilities
- it would be helpful to set some realistic goals regarding employment: employment advice, not just disability advice was required. This was especially so for the person under consideration, who had already done much to empower herself
- they would need to know what services existed, where services were, and how services related to one another. Workshop members felt that this was not the picture at present
- services should be accessible
- support should be given to people once they were in employment – it should not be confined to helping people find employment
- professional standards were necessary. Singled out here was the need for people in vocational rehabilitation services to be accountable to their organisation. The Employment Service in particular was criticised for failing in this regard
- there ought to be an organised complaints procedure so that people who feel they have been discriminated against – by the vocational rehabilitation services, employers or some other agent – can have official channels through which to seek redress

- the difficulty with benefit entitlements was highlighted. It is quite conceivable for a disabled person to find their income threatened if they seek employment
- financial stability was also recommended for the services themselves. One-year contracting was seen to militate against coherent and consistent progress
- disabled people themselves should be involved in the design of vocational rehabilitation services. This would help to get things right first time, and would make training more appropriate to needs
- recognition of achievement was required: the whole process of vocational rehabilitation ought to be one of confidence-building.

Workshop 2: A Leg Amputation

The second workshop dealt with the case of a forty-six-year-old who had had a leg amputation following a traffic accident. As in the first workshop, they felt that a service should be flexible and accessible, that those working in it should be well trained with good customer-care skills, that effective assessment should be provided, and that it was important to agree on goals with the client. The service should also set itself objectives, review its performance, and make adjustments accordingly. In addition, there was particular emphasis on the following:

- the need for a holistic approach – one should not just focus on the disability itself
- disability should be positively marketed
- quality was essential.

Workshop 3: A Psychotic Episode

In the third workshop participants were presented with a case study of a twenty-four-year-old who had undergone intensive psychological counselling after suffering an acute psychotic episode. In their analysis they, too, saw the importance of an individual, flexible and client-focused approach, of the need for good quality assessment, identification of options, and supportive counselling, and of the benefits of a holistic viewpoint that included consideration of the social, personal and family network. Furthermore, some choice for the person regarding who works with them should be considered.

Two other points specifically related to mental health were also raised. The first was that the issue of stigma was particularly relevant – it was suggested that normalisation within mainstream provision was very important. The second was that the question of when to intervene was problematical – timing was critical and, in the case study, seemed to have occurred too late.

Workshop 4: A Severe Depression

The fourth workshop looked at the case of a thirty-six-year-old who had suffered severe depression following severe stress at work. Reinforcing a now-familiar theme it was considered important that an accessible, visible, professional and individually-focused service should exist. As before, the value of a quality assessment and continuous support was highlighted and, as in Workshop 3, the advantages of bringing in the family were recognised.

There was also, however, a new idea: that the client must have their problem put in perspective and viewed in objective terms. Given this may be hard for someone who may be feeling angry and inadequate, the client needs not just a counsellor but an advocate. This advocate should, in addition, be a constant, i.e. one person throughout the rehabilitation process.

Workshop 5: Rheumatoid Arthritis

In Workshop 5 the case of a forty-one-year-old suffering from rheumatoid arthritis was assessed. As before, the group felt that a participative approach was crucial – it helped a person keep their dignity – and that professional empathy and an individual approach were vital. Once again they also felt that accessible, affordable help and goal-setting were important and, like Workshop 1, they pointed to the problems with benefits. Several other new points were raised, however:

- Access to peer groups could be very helpful. Clients should be targeted towards them, not just left to find them or stumble across them on their own
- There should be encouragement of self-help where appropriate
- Trust, confidentiality and impartial honesty were needed
- It is important to get the right balance between aspirations and abilities
- The service provided should be seamless and comprehensive
- Professionals should have help themselves, possibly from a professional lead body like those that exist in industry. Such an organisation could help set national standards, suggest objectives and goals and set clear guidelines, and generally provide the sort of professional training that is given in the commercial sector
- It is crucial that the rehabilitation services keep abreast of changing job opportunities – it is no use rehabilitating people for employment that has disappeared
- Co-ordinated research and evaluation is needed to avoid duplication and to aid exchange of information and ideas.

Workshop 6: A Progressive Visual Disability

The final workshop group investigated the case of a person with a progressive visual disability. In common with other groups they felt that the client should occupy the central position in the rehabilitation process, that they should feel in control, and that they should benefit from an individual approach. As in the fifth group the value of peer group support was mentioned. Continual exchange of information was also seen as helpful so that everyone could feel involved all the time.

Discussion in the Plenary Session

Donal McAnaney described how the City and Guilds Institute have introduced something called 'accreditation of prior learning', a process through which you can use all kinds of evidence to show skills relevant to employment – for example, running a family budget. The same principle, he felt, could be applied in the Employment Rehabilitation Service, where it could help people to put all their experiences in a positive work-related light.

Another participant explained how she has already been putting into practice much of what the workshops had suggested should be done. However, she also pointed out that, working for a charity, there are big problems in raising funding: without funding, of course, it is very difficult to put any good ideas into practice. And, as someone else said, in the current economic climate there are serious obstacles to implementing some of the prescriptions made in the Workshops.

A representative from the London Employment Service commented that in the Workshops much stress was laid on the need for practical training. He wanted to know where that sort of training is coming from now, and where it might come from in future. In response someone from the Employment Rehabilitation Service explained that part of the training will come from the new Ability Development Centres (ADCs), which will have trainers and a training manager. In addition people will continue to be trained at the national training centre in Manchester, which has recently been revamping and improving what it provides. There is also an expressed hope to work closely with voluntary organisations and organisations that are experienced in the care of people with disabilities, with the aim of co-hosting and facilitating training to get the best from everyone. ADC managers will of course be working together nationally to keep abreast of training activities.

On the same theme of training one delegate felt that in Britain people working in the disability field have not been recognised as a profession in their own right – unlike in the US. He thought that this country could make better use of European programmes. Progress is occurring, however: Brenda Smith pointed out that City University had just developed a new Master's course on 'Disability Management'.

Moving on to a different subject, it was argued that for most people with disabilities who have been out of work for some time, the best way back into employment is one step at a time via part-time work. However, all that exists at present is financially-limited sheltered placement schemes, therapeutic earnings and the new disability working allowance (which does not apply to anyone on therapeutic earnings or anyone claiming housing benefit). It was felt that this whole area really needed improvement – if there were more part-time opportunities there might be far more successful outcomes.

A new issue was also raised: the potential need for financial advice, both to guide clients through the benefits minefield and to try to assist people who may have suffered serious falls in income following disability.

In conclusion, the chairman reminded participants that while there were good reasons to focus on clients' needs and perspectives and to stress the advantages of an individual and flexible approach, one should not become obsessive about not categorising people. The planning and structuring of services is impossible without grouping and classifying people to some extent: therefore it was important not to be afraid of using such categories sometimes in thinking about, analysing and planning rehabilitation services.

PART II

A European Perspective

CHAPTER SIX

Maastricht and Vocational Rehabilitation

Donal McAnaney

Introduction

This chapter examines the impact of the Treaty of European Union on people with disabilities, and at the possible future direction in which services may develop over the next four to six years.

I should point out though that I come from Ireland and Ireland is an Objective One region within the European Community. In other words, as a region of economic disadvantage with 20 per cent unemployment, Ireland has been a net beneficiary of European Structural Funds since 1974. For this reason people in Ireland may be more aware of the impact of being part of the European Community than people in some other Member States.

Second, I am a psychologist and not a lawyer, and therefore any interpretation I make of the Treaty has to be viewed with that caveat. However, as actors in the field of vocational rehabilitation for people with disabilities, it is important that we all become more aware of the potential of the range of European Actions in favour of people with disabilities and how these may be influenced by the new treaty.

My interest in European Treaties arose from the Inaugural Conference of European Confederation for the Employment of People with Disabilities (CEEH) in Paris in 1990. At this conference it was proposed that Non-Governmental Organisations (NGOs) in Europe should pursue the adoption of a directive by the European Commission (EC) on the employment rights of people with disabilities similar to those protecting the rights of women on the workplace. [An EC Directive must be passed into law in the Member States within a specified time period.] With this in mind I began to examine the Treaty of Rome to understand how the system worked for women and how it might be operated on behalf of people with disabilities in order to achieve an EC directive on equal rights for people with disabilities.

I was rather disappointed when I read the Treaty of Rome to find that, in terms of social policy, the Treaty of Rome was very 'soft'. There was no provision for the Commission to issue directives on social policy apart from the equal-pay Article for women. The Commission's competence extended to promoting discussions, issuing recommendations, and facilitating research and funding vocational training, but it could not issue directives to the Member States on how to manage their own affairs in the area of social policy.

However, it was clear that the competence of the Commission could be broadened through amending the Treaty. For example, most people who voted for the Single European Act were probably unaware that they were also voting to give the Commission power to issue directives in the area of public health and safety. The effect of this amendment can be seen in every workplace in the European Community in terms of Safety Statements and Safety Officers, etc. It seemed to me that in any sphere in which the European Community has competence to act, it can be a useful agent for change. Unfortunately in the past the Commission has had no competence in any issues which are unrelated to the economy and the labour market. Consequently such areas as social rehabilitation, education and equal rights were only marginally effected under the Treaty of Rome.

The purpose of this chapter is to compare certain sections of the Treaty of Maastricht with the Treaty of Rome in order to tease out what changes may be on the horizon for people with disabilities. I will focus on certain important Articles in the new Treaty and compare the 1987 wording with the 1992 wording. In examining the wording of the Treaty the objective is to identify a possible window of opportunity that actors in the field of disabilities can start to push open to broaden rights and opportunities at both a national and a European level.

Table 6.1

1987	ARTICLE 2	1992
	Common Market	
Approximating Economic policy		Economic and Monetary Union
	Harmonious development of economic activity	
Continuous and balanced expansion		Sustainable and non-inflationary growth repecting the environment
Increase in Stability		Convergence of economic performance
Accelerated raising of the standard of living		High level of employment and *social protection* raising the standard of living and *quality of life*
		Economic and social cohesion
Closer relations between Member States		Solidarity among Member States

The Principles of the Treaty of European Union

Article 2 summarises the goals of European Union and as such is worth reviewing. A summary of the content is presented in Table 6.1 for reference. Both the 1987 and 1992 Articles refer to a common market, and harmonious development of economic activity. But in 1987 the focus was upon approximating economic policy, whereas the new Treaty refers to economic and monetary union. In 1987, a continuous and balanced expansion were the terms used, whereas Maastrict refers to sustainable and non-inflationary growth respecting the environment. An increase in stability in the 1987 Treaty becomes a convergence of economic performance in the 1992 version. An accelerated rise in the standard of living is reframed in the current Treaty as a high level of employment and social protection raising the standard of living and quality of life.

This brief analysis shows a substantial change in the philosophy underlying the Treaty of European Union. It is possible to see some 'softer' edges as in the references to the environment and quality of life but a much stronger emphasis on economic union and convergence, on economic and social cohesion and on solidarity among member states.

In general, I think there are some opportunities for promoting the rights of disabled people, especially in the area of improving quality of life. One must remember that the intent of an Article becomes transformed into action through the Commission by programmes, regulations and in many cases funding. So one cannot be completely certain of the intent of a particular Article until these have been implemented.

Table 6.2 gives a brief comparison of the policy objectives of Article 3 in both Treaties. In the 1987 and 1992 versions of Article 3 such things as the elimination of customs duties: common commercial policy; freedom of movement of goods, persons, services and capital; common agricultural policy; common transport policy; and the distortion of competition are addressed.

The approximation of laws in relation to the common market has also been included in both Treaties. This is an interesting detail to explore. It may appear, on the surface, that one could make a case that all Member States should harmonise employment legislation in relation to the employment of people with disabilities. However, this approximation of laws does not stretch to such legislation as, for example, Employment Quota/Levies for people with a disability. This was a 'cul de sac' which I followed up for a couple of months in relation to the Treaty of Rome. It transpires that national governments can impose upon themselves any laws they may wish but if such laws make them less competitive, there can be no requirement to harmonise.

The final elements in the 1987 Treaty were: the co-ordination of economic policies and a European Social Fund (ESF) to improve employment opportunities and raise the standard of living. This narrow definition of the focus of the European Social Fund meant that it was seen mainly as an instrument for labour market adjustments. Consequently, all ESF fundable activities had to have vocational training as the method and employment as the outcome regardless of the needs or abilities of those participating.

Table 6.2

1987	ARTICLE 3	1992
	Elimination of custom duties etc.	
	Common commercial policy	
	Freedom of movement of goods, persons, services and capital	
		Entry and movement of persons on Internal Market and fisheries
	Common policy in agriculture	
	Common policy in transport	
	Ensure competition is not distorted	
Coordination of economic policies		
	Approximation of laws in relation to Common Market	
European Social Fund to improve employment opportunities and raise standard of living		A policy in the social sphere comprising a European Social Fund
		Economic and social cohesion
		A policy in the sphere of the environment
		Strengthening competitiveness of community industry
		Promotion of research and technical development
		Trans-European Networks
		High level of Health Protection
		Education and Training of high quality and flowering of culture
		Policy in sphere of development
	An association of overseas countries	
		Consumer protection
		Energy, civil protection and tourism

In contrast the Treaty of Maastricht refers to a policy in the social sphere comprising the European Social Fund. This is very broad, and is left totally open for interpretation. In the short term, that is between now [1992] and 1997, nothing much will change. But it is a window which can be pushed in terms of improving the social conditions of people with disabilities. I will return to this in relation to Article 123 which deals directly with the Social Fund.

Other interesting changes relate to the specific mention of promotion of research and technical developments which will ensure the continuance of programmes such as TIDE (Technology Initiatives for the Disabled and Elderly). It may be possible also to promote social rehabilitation research as a valid research under the ESF. Such research can be grant aided up to 100 per cent of costs whereas in the normal course of events 'additionality' of Member States funding is required for activities.

Finally the specific references to education and culture should have a significant impact in the next few years. In the past funding for education was not available unless it was vocational in nature. Now, within these boundaries it would appear that developments in education will become eligible for funding.

European Citizenship

Prior to the Treaty, there was talk about citizenship and the specification of rights of individuals under European Law. CEEH, in addition to many other representative groups, formulated proposals for some changes to the Treaty that would have made people with disabilities entitled to a number of civil rights.

In fact the European Parliament recommended the following Article for inclusion in the Treaty: 'in the field of application of community law, everyone shall be equal before the law. Any discrimination on grounds such as race, colour, sex, language, religion, political or other opinions, national or social origin, association with a national minority, property, birth or other status shall be prohibited.'

One has to question why the European Parliament did not appear to be aware of disability when drafting this Article. I feel it is a comment on the efficacy of the Disability Lobby at a European level. We, who are actors in the field of disability, have to think about the fact that we are part of the Community and come together to influence developments more directly. The new Treaty has made it easier for us to do so, but easier does not mean less complicated, as I will discuss later.

In the event none of these suggestions were included in the Treaty despite the recommendation of the European Parliament. The citizenship chapter which finally emerged is summarised in Table 6.3. The rights conferred by the Treaty are these: the right to move freely between countries; the right to vote and stand as a candidate in any member state; municipal or European elections; the right to protection by the diplomatic authority or any member state wherever you are in the world; the right to petition the European Parliament; and the right to apply to an ombudsman. However, it has been left open so that other rights can be added or strengthened in the future and this is something that lobby groups and organisations of and for people with disabilities should keep an eye on when the next amendment to the Treaty is scheduled (probably around 1997).

Table 6.3 Citizenship of the Union

Rights conferred by Treaty – not clearly specified apart from:
- Right to move freely
- Right to vote and stand as a candidate in any Member State Municipal and European Elections
- Right to protection by the diplomatic authority of any Member State
- Right to petition European Parliament
- Application to Ombudsman

Rights can be added or strengthened

Social Policy, Education, Vocation Training and Youth

The 1987 title 'Social Policy' has been extended to include 'Social Policy, Education, Vocational Training and Youth'. While this indicates a change in priorities, little will change in reality between now and 1997.

This becomes obvious when one examines Table 6.4 which compares the seven key articles on social policy in their present format with the previous version. Apart from the way in which issues of health and safety are handled no changes have been made. This is possibly a result of the controversy over what is now known as the Social Protocol but which was originally intended as the Social Chapter. The reference to Article 189c under Health and Safety indicates a procedure by which an Act can be adopted. This procedure, which is an important element in the strategy for promoting change within the EC, is presented in summary in Figure 6.1 and will be discussed in detail later.

The European Social Fund, which is at the core of Social Policy, has changed little in its role, as can be observed in Table 6.5. In 1987 the focus was upon rendering the employment of workers easier and increasing geographical and occupational mobility within the Union. To these have been added facilitating adaptation to industrial changes and changes in production systems, particularly through vocational training and retraining. An example can illustrate the way in which this may affect the application of European Social Funding. Previously an individual who was in a declining industry would have to become unemployed before any funds could be allocate towards retraining. It would appear that the current position, in the case of someone in an industry that is facing major structural change, is that ESF can be applied to retraining while that person is still employed.

Table 6.4

1987	1992
Title III	*Title VIII*
Social Policy	*Social Policy, Education*
	Vocational Training & Youth

ARTICLE 117

Improvement of working conditions

Improved standard of living for workers

ARTICLE 118

Matters in the social field
- Employment
- Labour law and working conditions
- Basic and advanced Vocational Training
- Social Security
- Prevention of occupational accidents and diseases
- Occupational hygiene
- Right of Association & collective bargaining

ARTICLE 118A

Health & Safety

Directives for Minimum requirements	Procedure laid down in 189c

ARTICLE 119

Equal pay

ARTICLE 120

Paid holiday schemes

ARTICLE 121

Social Security for Migrant Workers

ARTICLE 122

Reports on progress

ADOPTION OF AN ACT

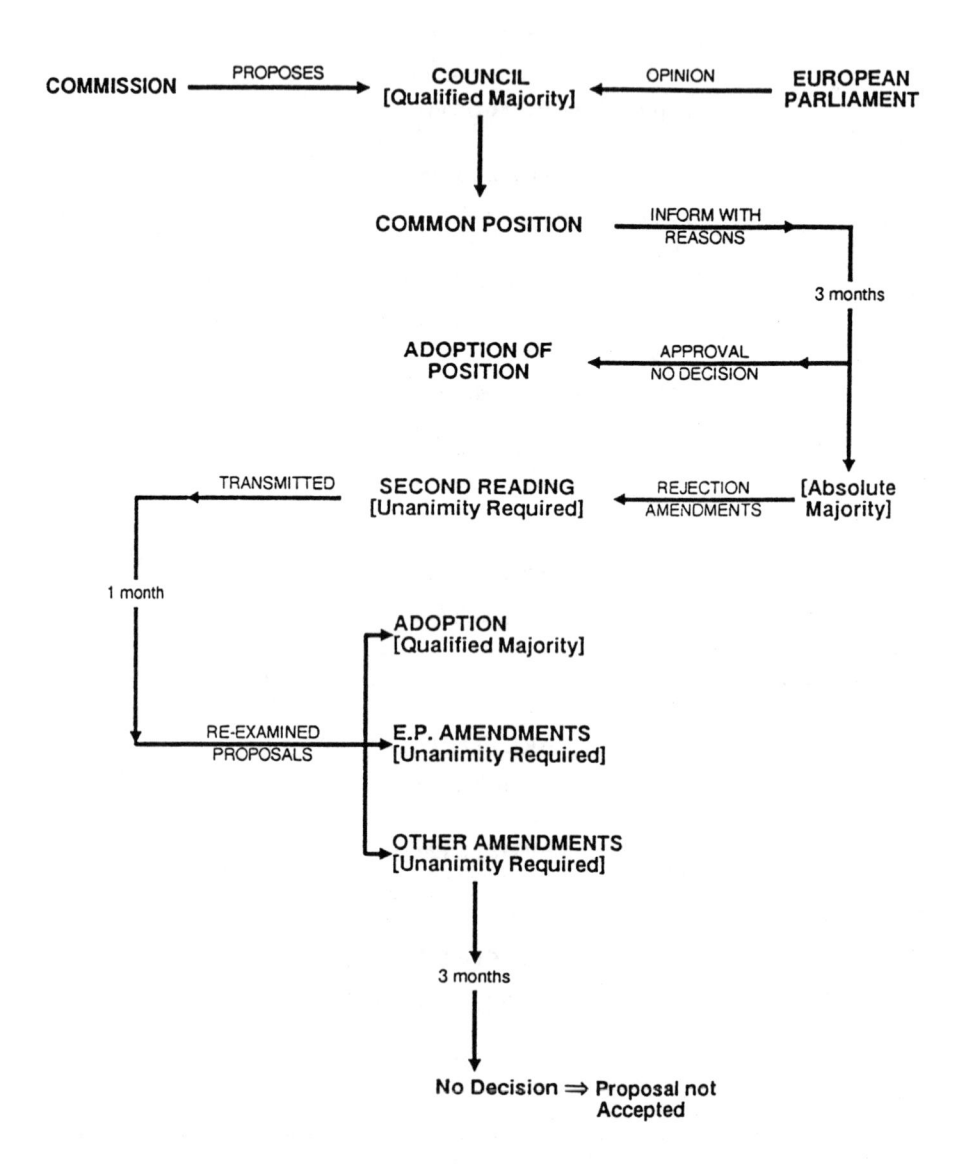

COMMISSION —PROPOSES→ COUNCIL [Qualified Majority] ←OPINION— EUROPEAN PARLIAMENT

↓

COMMON POSITION —INFORM WITH REASONS→

3 months

ADOPTION OF POSITION ←APPROVAL / NO DECISION—

[Absolute Majority]

SECOND READING [Unanimity Required] ←REJECTION / AMENDMENTS—

←TRANSMITTED—

1 month

↓ RE-EXAMINED PROPOSALS →

- ADOPTION [Qualified Majority]
- E.P. AMENDMENTS [Unanimity Required]
- OTHER AMENDMENTS [Unanimity Required]

3 months

↓

No Decision ⇒ Proposal not Accepted

Figure 6.1 Article 189c

Table 6.5 European Social Fund

1987	1992

ARTICLE 123

Render employment of workers easier

Increase geographical and occupational mobility within community

Facilitate adaptation to industrial changes and changes in production systems

Particular through Vocational Training and retraining

ARTICLE 124

Administration of fund by Commission

ARTICLE 125

50% of expenditure
Productive re-employment
- vocational retraining
- resettlement allowances

Council in accordance with procedure in Article 189c shall adopt implementary decisions relating to the European Social Fund

ARTICLE 126

Qualified majority –
Discontinuation of ESF

Unanimous –
Determination of new tasks

Education, Vocational Training and Youth

Development of quality education
- European dimension
- Mobility of teachers and students
- Cooperation between Educational Establishments
- Exchange of experiences and information
- Youth exchanges
- Distance Education

Incentive measures

Article 125 has been altered so that the focus or field of application of the European Social Fund can be changed without changing the Treaty. In 1992, the Council, in accordance with the procedures set down in Article 189C, shall adopt implementer decisions relating to the European Social Fund. This opens up possibilities for broadening the scope of the ESF. It means that, should the disability lobby develop an effective European advocacy, a change in emphasis within the Social Fund could be accomplished.

To convince the Council to adopt an implementer decision relating to the European Social Fund means going down a long road. No one country or no single small local group is likely to achieve such a goal. But I am optimistic that some kind of broadening of the field of application of the ESF could be achieved within the next five years. The important thing at the moment is the recognition that such a possibility exists and that there is a need to sit down together to establish a common platform in this area across all disability groups and all key actors in the field at a European level. It is not a question of whether progress can be achieved, but of how it should be achieved, and in which areas it could have the greatest impact for European citizens with disabilities.

Article 126 has been completely rewritten and, for the first time, refers to education. Specifically the Treaty outlines the areas of development of quality education with a European dimension, mobility of teachers and students, co-operation between educational establishments, exchange of experience and information, youth exchanges and distance education. It is difficult to comment further upon this until the level of funding which will be available under this heading and the regulations pertaining to it are published. However, it is an important development which must be monitored closely.

The Social Protocol

The objectives of the Social Protocol [Table 6.6] are the promotion of employment, improved living and working conditions, social protection, dialogue between management and labour, and the development of human resources. From the perspective of people with disability in Europe, the most significant aspect of the Social Protocol is the introduction of a new term: 'combating exclusion'.

The meaning of 'exclusion' has been debated vigorously both within and outside the Commission. The key concern is the breadth of application of the term. It can be interpreted to mean being excluded from the labour market in which case there will be many people who are currently marginalised who will not benefit from these measures. On the other hand 'social exclusion' in broader terms might also be addressed. Once again the deciding factors will be the degree of flexibility within the regulations and the level of funding for measures to combat exclusion. It is likely that such initiatives as HORIZON, NOW, and EUROFORM will form the model for the exclusion fund.

We can debate the desirability of introducing another term, 'the excluded', to the vocabulary of social and vocational rehabilitation as an alternative to 'disabled' or 'marginalised', but what is important is that exclusion has become a central concern within the European Parliament (EP) and a legitimate object for intervention by the Commission.

Table 6.6 Social Protocol

ARTICLE 1

Promotion of employment

Improved living and working conditions

Social Protection

Dialogue between management and labour

Development of human resources • high employment

• combat exclusion*

ARTICLE 2

1. Health & Safety
   Working Conditions
   Information and consultation of workers
   Equality between men and women
   * Integration of persons excluded from the labour market

2. Directives, minimum requirement for gradual implementation without undue burden on small and medium size undertakings Article 189c Procedures

3. Unanimous Action on:
   - Social Security and Social Protection
   - Protection of workers where employment is terminated
   - Representation and collective defence of workers and employers
   - Conditions of employment for 3rd country nationals
   - Financial contributions for employment and job creation

4. Management and labour entrusted with implementation Does not apply to right of association, right to strike and the right to impose lock-outs

Promoting Change: Procedures for the Adoption of an Act

The means by which the EP can alter the direction, intention or field of application of a number of crucial policies and instruments has been specified in Article 3. This Article has been referred to a number of times during the course of this paper in relation to Health and Safety and the ESF.

The adoption of an act under the Maastricht Treaty requires a qualified majority at the Council of Ministers of a common position which is either approved by the EP or upon which no decision has been reached by the EP. However, should the EP reject, or suggest amendments, a unanimous decision of the Council is required in order to progress further. In the event that this is achieved the Commission must resubmit an amended proposal to the Council, taking into account the views of the EP, which can accept the re-examined proposal by a qualified majority or further amend it by a unanimous decision.

One interesting aspect of this procedure is the 'statute of limitations' on each of the phases. These are respectively: three months for the European Parliament to respond to the Council's common position, one month for the Commission to respond to the second reading, and three months for the Council to make its final decision. If such a decision has not been reached within the time limit, the proposal is deemed not to be accepted.

The message for a European Disability lobby should be clear. Not only is it essential that a common position be agreed between all actors in the disability field, including organisations of and for people with disabilities, but this common position must be clearly and concisely communicated, and support obtained, at a regional, a national and a European parliamentary level.

In addition, once the process has been activated, a high level of energy, effort and constant monitoring of the process will be required to ensure that the deadlines are met by the various institutions involved. Hypothetically, a proposal could reach the final hurdle and be pushed off the agenda of the Council of Ministers by some international crisis. In this event the process would have to be restarted from scratch.

Given the evident lack of success of the European Disability Lobby during the Maastricht process, it is unlikely that such a major task could be undertaken at the present time. However, the opportunity for developing consensus within the field of disability is available and must be acted upon. A first step in this direction is the raising of awareness amongst local, regional, national and European actors in the field of disability of the possibility of positive action within the context of the Treaty of European Union.

Implications for the Future

There are two ways to see into the future. One can either resort to the science of futurology, which creates models to predict future trends, or apply the techniques of the science of astrology. I have decided to use astrology as the most suitable metaphor for characterising the way ahead. I have constructed an 'astrological chart' for disability services from which one may project into the future. Many of the issues which have been discussed throughout the conference feature on this chart. Firstly, there are the constellation of issues which are currently impinging on the nature of services for people with disabilities.

Service Quality

We have heard reference to the British Standard for Service Quality BS 5750. ISO 9004 is the international standard equivalent. It is only a guideline at the moment but it will become a standard for service quality. Quality Service Systems will eventually be installed in airlines, in banks, in BT, in order to accredit their services in terms of quality. Previous standards have been production-based and so their application to services for people with disabilities resulted in a kind of dehumanising of the person or the focus of the service because consumers tended to be characterised as stock or product. But ISO 9004 looks specifically at services to people and personal services.

Some progress towards a quality system has been made in Ireland over the past two years. The National Rehabilitation Board has agreed standards with the actors in the field of vocational training for people with disabilities. For example, standard number one lays down that any organisation wishing to offer a vocational service to people with disabilities must have a mission statement. The mission statement must clearly state the goals of the organisation. Standard number two requires that an intention to enable and empower people with disabilities must be explicit in that mission statement. These are just two ideas of the way in which service quality and service quality systems will affect delivery in the future.

Monitoring and Evaluation

These were also referred to during the course of the conference. Monitoring and evaluation are well established as part of the service delivery system in the United States. The European Commission has recently carried out a major evaluation of the use of funds in the European Community for people with disabilities which was implemented in all 12 Member States. Within the next Community Support Programme and Community Initiative Programme evaluation and monitoring at both a national level and at a European level will become a crucial precondition for the receipt of funds. From the perspective of the disability field it is important that evaluation is not based on purely quantitative information; there are many qualitative issues which must be taken on board as well.

Rights Legislation

This is another issue which has been raised. I believe that Rights Legislation can, and will, be implemented over the next ten years. It is likely that it will take the form of Anti-Discrimination Legislation, mainly because this has the lowest cost implications for national governments. Getting the legislation in place is only the first step in achieving equal rights for people with disabilities. The second step is training to implement legislation which has been passed. This has proved much more difficult in relation to the Act, sponsored by Tom Clarke, than one would have expected.

Special Needs Focus

My own view is that we must move away from what I term 'disability box' terminology – people being blind, people being deaf, people being mentally ill, etc. – and move towards a special needs focus which concentrates on the person first rather than their disability. This approach has been adopted with indifferent effect in the Education Act and is included in the Tom Clarke Act. Basically such legislation will specify that a person in entitled to a statement of his or her needs and place a statutory responsibility on some authority to provide for those needs. In this way legislation can help us to move away from labelling and categorisation.

Multi-Disciplinary Delivery

As a step towards de-labelling and de-stigmatising the consumers of services, we must stop categorising ourselves and boxing ourselves as professionals. The professional boundaries and demarcations we create between ourselves foster the factionalisation of the person. It may be comfortable but it is no longer acceptable to say, 'I am responsible for your arm or leg, your home circumstances and emotional well-being are someone else's business. This narrow interdisciplinary approach is limited the things that can be achieved. The response is the development of a multidisciplinary delivery system where the team are sharing skills and experience and where the client is able to access whatever he or she feels is required from one source.

Client-Centred Ethos

A multidisciplinary delivery system is more congruent with a client-centred ethos. Every other presenter at the conference made reference to this. HELIOS I convened a conference in 1990 in Brussels where there were representatives of 50 centres from all over Europe and representatives of all the Local Model Activities as well. The objective of this seminar was to review the UN Declaration from the Year of the Disabled, the ILO Conventions on employing people with disabilities, and the Council of Europe recommendation on employment and training for people with disabilities. Each document had been published around 1984 or 1985. One common conclusion of the seminar was that the language in which the documents were written was inappropriate, or it had a professional bias. For example, under the heading 'Assessment' a handicapped person had the right to be assessed by the appropriate experts using the most up-to-date techniques. There was a general consensus which was virtually trans-European that the language and the philosophy had to change. However, there can be inertia in achieving such change. It is easier to claim to be a client-centred service than to deliver one. As service providers we should look at our approaches and methodologies before somebody else does it for us.

New Technology

We have not seen the end of the impact of New Technology. It will continue to impact strongly on services and employment. As it is, many of the services which are provided are becoming irrelevant and out of date in relation to open industry. New Technology impacts upon the disability field in at least five major domains. These domains stretch from instructional technology and access technology to applications, production and information management technologies. The pace of change in these fields means that every organisation will require a dedicated New Technology expert to update what is available and advise on new equipment.

Community-Based Services

Services are tending to become community-based and there is a trend in the Health sector away from larger institutions. This may be seen as a threat by some but it opens the opportunity to try and solve some old problems using new solutions. The inherent danger in any community-based strategy is the reduction of resources that seems to be implicit in such strategies from a fiscal perspective. This can be avoided by larger institutions and centres proactively promoting community-based options for their clients.

Integration

The pro and cons of the integration debate have been well argued within the sphere of special education. As with community-based strategies, the issue hinges around resourcing. Specialist services will always have their place in the development of people with disabilities but the important move must be from closed rehabilitation systems to more open systems. To quote a tenet of Italian rehabilitation, 'We train people in order to integrate them, why don't we integrate people to train them?' A wide variety of creative and flexible options will have to be created in order to meet the needs of people with disabilities. These options must range from highly supported and resourced contexts to low support open environments. In addition, the individual must be facilitated to move easily from one option to another with the minimum of bureaucracy.

The above issues do not impact directly upon people with disabilities. They pervade the debate between funders and providers, people with disabilities and advocates and between the many interest groups in the field. They impact through the real world of services for people with disabilities. For this reason I have included in the lower half of Figure 6.2 a schematic representation of the major actors in the field of disability in Europe and how they interrelate.

This representation characterises service providers as contractors. This is the way service provision is being viewed. Contracting will become more and more common over the next five years. In European terms automatic annual funding has given way to a system of programming over two to three years. National governments will probably start to move into a similar type of approach. Funding will be allocated to certain programmes for a set period of time on the basis of agreed costs and benefits.

Given the complexity of the relationships, clear communication between actors is a priority. There will be funding between the European Commission and national governments, funding from national governments, funding from regional governments. The whole idea of subsidiarity is to give more power to the regions. So, for instance, Strathclyde Regional Council, which actually has the same population as the Republic of Ireland, would have the same kind of mandate from Europe in terms of subsidiarity to work for their population.

All Member States governments will be funding consumer organisations within the next five years. These consumer organisations can be extremely important and effective lobby groups and will be looking very closely at the service provided to them through the current system. Their criticisms and demands will have to be taken on board. Service providers should be participat-

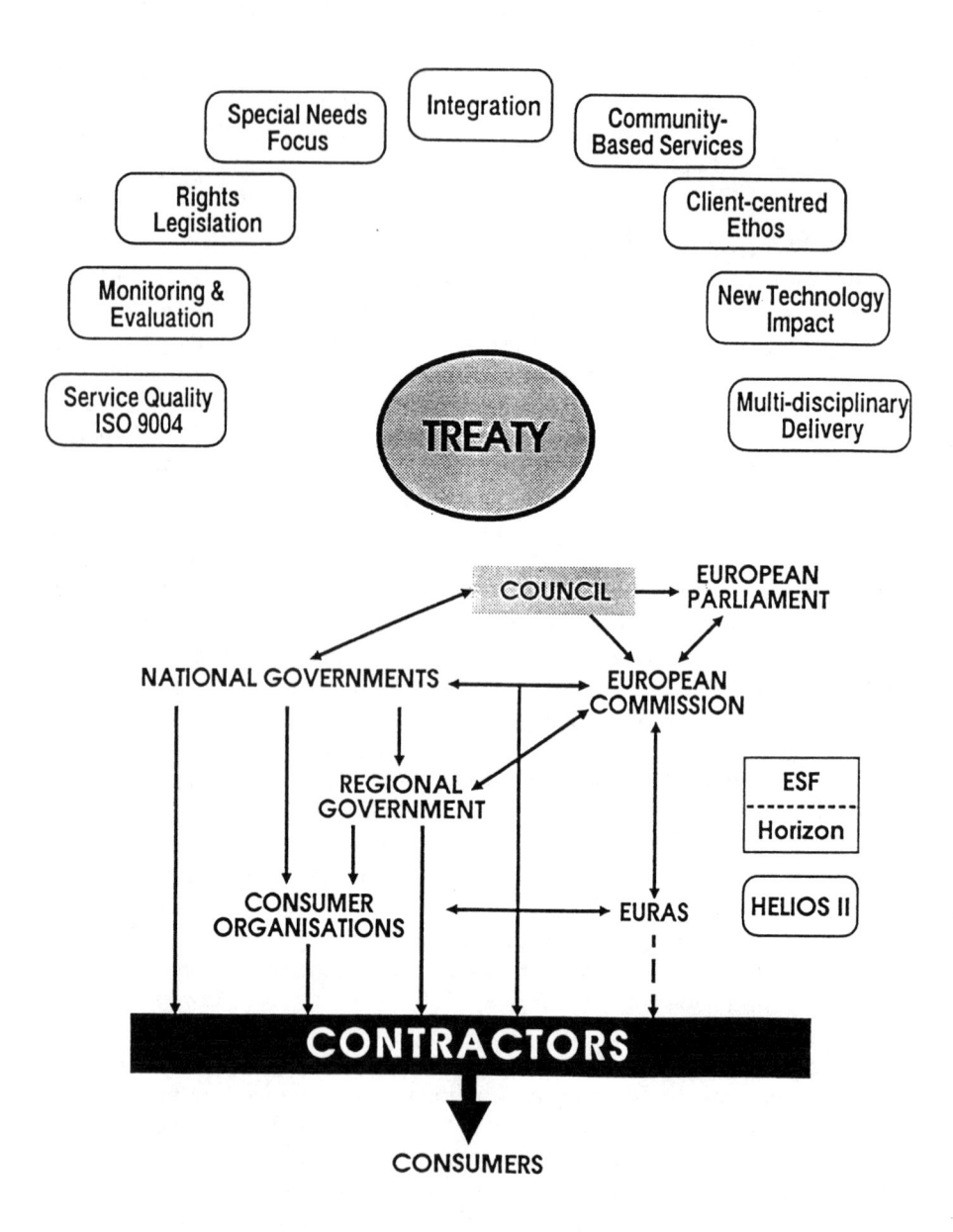

Figure 6.2

ing with these organisations in planning the future direction of services in order to achieve greater relevance and consumer satisfaction. Finally, the European Commission, through HELIOS II programme, is funding European NGOs (non-governmental organisation). These are likely to become more vocal and more effective in promoting the views of people with disabilities to the Commission. Their views will be taken on board in the development of any new programmes and regulations in the disability field.

At the bottom of Figure 6.2 the word 'consumer' has been placed in order to indicate the status that people who must use services are assigned at the moment. The task for the future is to move from the constellation of special issues, through the opportunities provided under the new Treaty, through the complex systems and structures of policy-making, service provision and funding, and actually deliver a more flexible, open, accountable and human service to the individual.

In order to achieve this we, as actors in the field of disability, have to become involved in a collective advocacy. It would appear that this approach has born fruit in the United States in terms of the Americans with Disabilities Act. The National Council for Voluntary Organisations (NCVO) is a particularly good example of how this can work. They have become very aware of the way things are developing. They know what is going on. They are a very useful organisation and very impressive in terms of their knowledge and their intention to support voluntary agencies.

We now have five years in which to work together in collective advocacy towards the next opportunity to effect European legislation. In Ireland one response to this challenge has been the formation of the Irish Council for Training, Development and Employment for People with Disabilities. It embraces all disabilities, service providers and people with disabilities themselves with the sole goal of promoting the full participation and equal access of people with disabilities in training and employment opportunities. I think this ties in with what Frank Coffield calls 'partnership' rather than 'competition'.

In the normal course of events, organisations of and for people with disabilities have been in competition for finance and political influence. But this lets the funders and policy makers off the hook. One interest group can be played off against the next. If all actors in the field can come together around a common platform, it may be possible actually to increase the overall budget for people with disabilities, achieve appropriate legislation and improve services.

CHAPTER SEVEN

Lessons from the First Horizon Programme

Erwin Seyfried

The Horizon Group of Experts

This group was formed at the end of 1992. Its aim was to monitor the implementation of the programme at European Commission level, making proposals on the methodology and organisation of its evaluation and of advising the Commission on its preparation of the new Community Initiatives in the field of human resources for the period from 1994 to 1999.

It was active until the end of 1993 and consisted of seven individuals whose varying backgrounds and experiences covered the target groups affected by the Horizon Programme.

However it is not easy to look at the future of Community Initiatives. The lack of synchronisation in the course of the transnational programme highlights one of the many problems experienced in the implementation of the Horizon programme, problems which had to be considered by the Experts Group in order to submit proposals for their solution to the European Commission. In the case of this lack of synchronisation our proposal for the next Initiative was that there should be a fixed deadline for the approval of local projects, binding for all member states.

I only wish to deal with such problems to the extent that it is possible to draw conclusions for the future of the Community Initiatives. And it is this subject on which I shall therefore concentrate.

The 1993 Reform of the European Social Fund

In this context I would like to start by looking at the reform of the European Social Fund (ESF) which took place in July 1993, as it is this reform which provided the definition of the parameters which will also apply to the new Community Initiatives.

At the beginning of 1993 the Group of Experts was able, with the aid of previous experiences made with Horizon, to formulate initial recommendations for the reform of the Social Fund, recommendations which were then submitted to the Commission. What did these recommendations look like? In order to answer this question it is necessary to take a closer look at the course and at some of the results of the Horizon Programme. What were the specific characteristics of the programme, and what effects did they have? What conclusions can we draw?

In contrast with the mainstream Social Fund, Horizon was first of all a transnational programme. In reality Horizon's transnational dimension was pretty weak. In most cases transnationality did not form a key factor in programme and project planning. Most of the planning took local projects as its starting point, projects which were then supplemented by a transnational component in accordance with the funding regulations. Only when the funded projects were checked did it emerge that merely a small part of the funding was going into transnational activities, with the local project work taking up the lion's share of the budget. Hence the expectations about Horizon's results at the level of transfer of know-how can also be correspondingly low. I will come back later to the conclusions concerning these transnational aspects.

At local level, however, Horizon was a big step forward. The programme has brought about an extension of the target groups and the possible actions for their social and vocational promotion. Thus, for example, it is within the framework of Horizon that training for trainers has for the first time been explicitly and officially recognised as an eligible measure. In this respect Horizon has also differentiated for the first time between physical and mental disabilities. It is also worth noting that the German version of the communication to the member states, which publicly announced the Horizon Programme and which was published in the Official Journal of the European Communities of December 1991, also specifically stressed that persons with psychiatric disabilities should be seen as a target group in their own right. In other words the member states were called upon to plan differentiated actions, i.e. actions suited to the differing needs of the individual target groups.

Following the official communications further, we can see that eligible measures in favour of the people with disabilities can also be carried out in sheltered environments. Particularly in the Objective One regions of the Union, projects are to be promoted which can help improve the access of disabled and disadvantaged people to training and vocational opportunities. This means that Horizon also offered the possibility of improving the social preconditions for vocational integration, which often represent a greater barrier than the individual's disabilities.

This also applies, to a considerable extent, to the measures in favour of migrants, who have up till now received no consideration as a separate group in any of the specific programmes of the European Union. Horizon was the first serious attempt at a European policy in favour of the social and vocational integration of this group.

All these measures eligible in the Horizon framework represent a qualitative extension of the funding spectrum of the mainstream Social Fund. This extension was very enthusiastically received by the people 'on the ground', i.e. the local promoters, who also grasped its differentiated quality, which helped create the conditions necessary in order to do better justice to the complex requirements of disabled and socially disadvantaged people.

Building on this assessment of the qualitative modifications of the Social Fund brought about by Horizon, the Group of Experts attempted to draw relevant conclusions for the reform of the Structure Fund which took place in July 1994. Our recommendations to the Commission were as follows: if the Commission seriously wishes to support the vocational integration of groups with major social problems, then the course taken by Horizon should also be pursued vigorously in the future. The key words in our recommendation were:

- The eligible measures should be made even more flexible in order to have a genuine effect on the requirements of the target groups. On the level of the individual's flexibility of interventions this means leading the participants step by step towards the vocational sector and employment. The starting point for each activity should be the present situations and the special needs of the individuals concerned.
- A successful approach for vocational training and integration should include a further element: it should let the excluded persons themselves become the agents of social change. It is mainly the involvement in the shaping of one's own living conditions which creates chances for personal development leading to autonomy. Every form of training needs the active participation of the individuals affected in this act of shaping. Activities for the development of training methodologies and measures based on self-autonomous approaches and including the acquisition of basic skills as well as the provision of supportive social relationships should thus be encouraged.
- There can be no doubt that, at the individual level, the improvement of skills and qualifications is an important precondition for social and vocational integration. On the other hand, there can equally be little doubt that this precondition is in itself insufficient. Vocational qualifications are useless if they cannot be used inside the labour market. Therefore it is necessary to create doors for entry into employment. Overcoming exclusion has to be enacted on two levels; the development of individual potential should be accompanied by the overcoming of barriers which constitute exclusion and by the creation of employment possibilities. A new Community Initiative against exclusion from the labour market makes all the more sense, the more it addresses this dual task.
- The description of the target groups for the ESF's new Objective Three should take into consideration the difficult starting conditions faced by socially excluded groups, who often have a long way to go before we can think of vocational integration into the general labour market.

When I came to read the final text of the new regulations on the Social Fund much later, I was quite delighted. I presume that many persons and authorities have contributed to them. Nevertheless, as you may have read yourselves, they essentially follow the lines that was taken by the Group of Experts. The ESF's field of activity has indeed been extended, and the key sentence in the new regulations for the ESF Objective Three is: 'explicit attention is to be paid to persons threatened by exclusion from the labour market and the selection criteria for categories already deemed eligible are to be made more flexible'.

Of course the central focus of a labour market policy instrument such as the ESF has to be a vocational qualification; yet in the new regulation concerning the groups we are interested in, the emphasis on vocational training is on an equal footing with the emphasis placed on career guidance, motivation and counselling measures or with the emphasis on the teaching of basic skills.

This extension of the measures relating to the individual person is supplemented in the new ESF regulation, by measures on the structural level directed towards 'the development of suitable training, employment and support structures, and the provision of facilities for the care of persons who may require it.' This means that the ESF's range of potential applications has indeed been decisively enlarged and moved in the direction of employment.

With regard to the Community Initiatives our analysis of the programme and its course came to the conclusion that the transnational or European dimension of the programme had been inadequately defined, in spite of the fact that transnationality was intended to form the actual core of the Community Initiatives. I mentioned this weakness on the transnational level at the beginning. Neither the ESF regulations nor the communications to the member states concerning the Community Initiatives contain any further details on this topic.

Most of you will therefore agree with me when I say that the transnational co-operation between the member states can hardly be said to have been well planned – the lack of sychronisation in the running of the programme which I mentioned already is just one example of this – and thus the transnational partnerships between the local actors have also all too often occurred as the result of trial and error.

According to the recommendations made by the Group of Experts, the reform of the Social Fund ought to reinforce and provide better clarification of the transnational element of the Community Initiatives. Yet it cannot and indeed should not be the task of the Commission to define the aims of the co-operation between the member states. This must remain the task of the member states themselves. The European Commission can however stimulate this co-operation by means of the appropriate instructions.

In the context of the programmes which have taken place up till now, it was for example the national co-ordinators who have been an important, if not the most important instrument for promoting co-operation between the member states. Now, following Article 29a of regulation 2084/93, an administrative committee for the Community Initiatives has been set up to further reinforce this instrument and the role of the member states. The main actor is thus not only the Commission, rather it is the member states who are to take an important role in the creation of transnational activities, something which was not always clear in the past.

The new regulations contain a further paragraph on the Community Initiatives. This does however represent a doubtful advance compared with the old regulations, and that precisely with regard to transnationality. A new addition to this paragraph is a clause enabling two or more member states to make a joint application for funding to the Commission when actions of transnational interest are concerned.

The possibilities laid down in the new regulations for joint operational programmes between several member states are, in my opinion, thoroughly impracticable, given the current state of European integration, where the member states are jealously guarding the amount of money being made available to them. Who are the funds to go to, when two or more member states hand in a joint operational programme to the Commission? Who will raise the national co-financing?

Conclusions for the New Community Initiatives

It should be borne in mind at this point that not all ideas on the subject of transnationality can be dealt with at the level of the Social Fund regulations. It was not new regulations dealing specifically with the Community Initiatives which were passed last July, but rather a regulation which affects the Fund as a whole.

Many of the things concerning the Community Initiatives and transnationality can also be dealt with 'below' the level of the official regulations. The main thing is that these concerns do get dealt with, which seems too often not to be the case, as we have already seen in the lack of synchronicity in the running of the programme. What are the main issues which should be clarified?

Transnationality

A transnational programme must take transnationality as the starting point of its ideas and planning, and at the end there should also above all be some recognisable added value for the Community.

The first step towards guaranteeing this should consist of the Commission considerably raising the funding for preparatory technical assistance for the member states, hence making possible a joint planning phase, which should also receive due consideration in the schedule for the running of the programme itself.

A phase of this sort could allow the member states to define fields of a common interest and requirements for joint action, whether with regard to particular measures or particular target groups, before and independently of the concrete local project applications. Building further on this it might then be possible to determine potential fields of transnational co-operation between local projects.

A checklist should also be drawn up for local projects intending to enter into transnational partnerships. The checklist should ensure that the partners are pursuing the same objectives and interests and are directed towards the same target groups. In addition the object and methods of transational co-operation should in the future be more clearly defined than has often been the case up till now. Co-operation does not mean that all the partners do the same thing, but rather that each one makes a specific contribution towards a common goal. To facilitate orientation in the difficult terrain of transnational co-operation, the Commission could produce a model agreement for co-operation between local partners.

Innovation

Something similar applies to the aim of trying to use the Community Initiatives to provide priority funding to innovative projects. Horizon and the other initiatives were also started with the intention of supporting innovative projects in particular. Yet in a similar way to the field of transnationality, what was actually to be understood by the term 'innovative' remained undefined.

In practice Horizon without a doubt helped in achieving considerable advances as compared with the mainstream Social Fund, which is of course used by many member states primarily as a means of refinancing their national labour market policies. Horizon's wide variety of funded projects seems to have given greater prominence to the programme's innovative aspects. The funding of local projects provided an important step in the direction of innovation, even if this step cannot be regarded as sufficient. For the question as to whether and to what extent certain local projects really can be said to be innovative remains largely unanswerable in terms of subjective assessments. In other words, criteria against which the term 'innovation' itself can be measured still have to be defined by the commission of the member states. In this context it is possible that such criteria for innovation could themselves provide a contribution to raising the quality of the programme, given that they could help local promoters in checking, modifying and developing further their own project ideas.

A more in-depth discussion about criteria and the function of innovation could perhaps prevent the results of innovative projects from evaporating without any long-term, structural effects being achieved, as has hitherto often been the case. This should at least be borne in mind, for it seems worse than senseless to promote local pilot schemes without thinking about how the results of such projects are to be taken up and developed further.

Conclusion

The European Parliament, whose powers have been somewhat – if insufficiently – increased by the treaty of Maastricht, has given the Commission a number of instructions concerning the Community Initiatives. The Parliament has recognised in principle the significance of the Community Initiatives and has even declared itself in favour of devoting 15 per cent of the entire Structure Fund budget to the Community Initiatives. The regulations of July 1993 fail however to follow these recommendations, and envisage only 9 per cent of the Structure Fund budget being allocated to the Community Initiatives.

In addition the European Parliament has also demanded that the number of Community Initiatives be significantly reduced, in order to simplify the administrative procedures and structures.

Current considerations in Brussels were tending towards creating a single Community Initiative in the field of Human Resources with a number of different emphases. It is however a matter of central importance that any such initiative should continue with the priorities set by Horizon. One of the great advantages of the Horizon Programme was the fact that it was clearly identifiable with regard to the target group intended to profit by it. As sensible as the European Parliament's demand to cut the number of Community Initiatives may be, it nevertheless remains just as necessary on the other hand for particularly disadvantaged groups to receive special attention, which is why the new Community Initiatives should also contain a clear commitment to prioritising action in their favour.

Throughout Europe Horizon has become well known as a specific programme for the handicapped, the socially disadvantaged and migrants, and has thus also helped create a new awareness for the needs of this group. For the sake of continuity it seems to me indispensable to extend this level of awareness which has been achieved. This would also mean keeping the well-marketed brand name Horizon for the corresponding priority areas within the new Community Initiatives.

CHAPTER EIGHT

The Helios Programme

Elizabeth Chennell

The European Union and Disability

All Member States of the European Union have a long tradition of policy actions directed towards improving employment opportunities for people with disabilities. These include quota schemes: support for employment rehabilitation centres and sheltered employment, provision of special aids, and codes of good practice for employers. But many of the underlying problems still remain. The following is a brief outline of the action taken by the European Union to support the policies of, and action by the Member States.

The European Union's approach is that people with disabilities should have the same opportunities as others. This was expressed in the Community Charter of the Fundamental Social Rights of Workers – The Social Charter, which was agreed to by all member States other than Britain. Article 28 of the Charter states that: 'All disabled persons, whatever the origin or nature of their disability, must be entitled to additional concrete measures aimed at improving their social and professional integration. These measures must concern, in particular, according to the capacities of the beneficiaries, vocational training, ergonomics, accessibility, mobility, means of transport and housing.' The general aim is 'to help people with disabilities to become capable of leading a normal independent life, fully integrated into society'.

This policy has been confirmed in the recent European Union white paper on Social Policy.

Objectives Concerning Employment for Disabled People

However, more specific objectives can generally be regarded as applying to policy and action in relation to employment:
- First, that people with disabilities should have facilities which are comparable to those for other people in their own country
- Second, that as far as possible, people with disabilities should work alongside people without disabilities
- Third, that people with disabilities and their representatives should be involved at all levels in programmes affecting them

- Fourth, that information about good practice should be disseminated widely within the Member States.

A number of specific initiatives have been undertaken.

Advice to Member States

The first concerned advice and commendations to Member States. In March 1981 a Resolution of the European Parliament stressed the need to promote the economic, social and vocational integration of disabled people. This was followed in 1986 by the adoption by the Council of Ministers of a Recommendation on the employment of disabled people. The Recommendation asserted that disabled people have the same right as all other workers to equal opportunity in training and employment, that in a period of economic crisis, action at European Community levels to promote the achievement of equal opportunity by means of positive and coherent policies should not only be continued but also intensified; and that these policies should take account of the aspirations of disabled people to a fully active and independent life.

It was also recommended to Member States that they should take all appropriate measures to promote fair opportunities for disabled people in the field of employment and vocational training, including initial training and employment as well as rehabilitation and resettlement.

The Commission responded to the 1988 Recommendation in a report to the Council. This report included descriptions of the position on legislation and provision for the employment of people with disabilities in each of the Member States. It was the first time that such an analysis had been made of the comparative situations in this area of activity.

The Council of Ministers stated its position on the Commission's report in its Conclusions of 12 June 1989. It considered that employment for disabled people must essentially be achieved through the implementation of general policies based on economic growth and job creation. The Council also considered that employment is an active social policy. Finally, the Council decided that the aim of measures to increase equal opportunities should first be to guarantee that no citizen of the European Union suffers discrimination with regard to access to vocational training or employment.

Action Programmes

The second area of activity centres on a series of action programmes which began in 1982. These initially focused on networks of rehabilitation centres. This was followed by the first HELIOS Programme in which much of the activity in relation to employment was centred on the networks of vocational training and rehabilitation centres, and subsequently by HELIOS II.

Improved Access

The third major area is improved access for people with disabilities for action on issues which are of concern to them. For instance, the European Social Fund provides financial support for major training initiatives. In addition, the principle aim of the HORIZON strand of the new EMPLOYMENT initiative is to improve access for disabled people to the labour market.

HELIOS II

The HELIOS II Programme started in 1993 and is due to run until the end of 1996. Vocational training, employment rehabilitation and economic integration are among the areas to be covered by HELIOS II. Certain priority themes have been identified for attention. These include information and advice for employers and trade unions; training methods and qualifications: transition from sheltered employment to open employment; and self-employment. It is also an essential feature of HELIOS II that co-operative action should be developed with non-governmental organisations (NGOs) of or for disabled

The Commission has no further specific proposals for legislation relating to the employment of disabled people. Any further initiatives will need to reflect the outcome of the work of HELIOS II and the results of the updating of the 1988 report on employment prepared by the Commission and Member States in 1987.

The HELIOS II Programme was born at the beginning of 1993 as the successor to HELIOS I. Its purpose is to promote integration and equal opportunities for all disabled people in the Union. Links between Member States which developed during the HELIOS I Programme continue to be fostered. But at the same time, new areas of co-operation and the more efficient pooling of practical information are needed.

With this in mind, one innovation of HELIOS II over HELIOS I is that the scope of the programme has been extended to include functional rehabilitation. In addition, action on integrated education will now encompass pre-school, higher and further education. These new areas, together with vocational training and employment rehabilitation, social and economic integration and independent living, form the framework for national measures supported by the Commission.

Annual Themes

The Council Decision of 25 February 1993 establishing the HELIOS II Programme provided that the exchange and information activities should be organised on specific annual themes. After consulting Member States' governments, NGOs, and Social Partners, the advisory bodies of the HELIOS II Programme themes were selected in seven areas. These included prevention, functional rehabilitation, education, social integration and independent living, social, economic and legal protection, and staff training. A number of priority themes and sub-themes are listed under each heading.

HELIOS II provides a framework for further co-operation with the HORIZON initiative on occupational rehabilitation and employment, and with the TIDE (Technology Initiatives for the Disabled and Elderly) initiative on the use of efficient technologies.

Moreover disabled people will be encouraged to take part in other Community programmes, particularly in the areas of training and preparation for working life, new technologies, vocational training and employment, equal opportunities for women and men, foreign language learning and youth exchanges within the Community.

Greater efforts to distribute information and raise public awareness regarding the possibilities for integrating disabled people form a major part of the HELIOS II Programme. The Commission has extended the scope of its co-operation with NGOs. The national disability councils and nationally representative NGOs are of great importance for the national co-ordination of activities. In addition, European NGOs and national disability councils give advice on specific questions relating to disability and integration as members of a newly established consultative body, the European Disability Forum.

NGO Activities in 1995

Following consultation with the European Disability Forum and the Advisory Committee, the Commission has approved the EURO-programmes drawn up by the Euro NGOs (European Non-Governmental Organisations) on the basis of the priority themes selected for HELIOS. These programmes may include conferences, seminars, study visits, training courses, meetings and other innovative European co-operation activities. The aims of these activities must correspond to the aims of the HELIOS Programme, namely: to promote equal opportunities for integration of disabled people. Commission assistance can cover a maximum of 50 per cent of eligible costs for approved activities, subject to a specified limit.

The 1995 EURO-programmes covered over 250 European activities. They were drawn up by the 12 Euro NGOs belonging to the European Disability Forum on the basis of applications for assistance submitted by national organisations and institutions before 1 November 1994. The various regions and the range of areas of disability are represented in the EURO-programmes that have been awarded Commission co-financing.

National HELIOS Information Days

Transnational exchange and information activities involve partners designated by the Member States. But information has to be circulated at national, regional and local level as well – hence the decision to organise national information days each year in all the Member States as part of the HELIOS II Programme, with financial support from the commission. The task of organising these events falls to the respective governments, with the co-operation of the national disability councils. The participants are chiefly partners in the activities of the HELIOS Programme, NGOs of disabled people, politicians, and representatives of the professions concerned, the authorities and the media.

CD-ROM HANDYNET

HANDYNET is one of the principal planks of the HELIOS Programme. It is a computerised information system and network for disabled people in Europe. The data is stored on CD-ROM, obviously vital given the importance of new technologies for the integration of disabled people.

The eighth version of CD-ROM HANDYNET became available in early 1995. Three hundred copies were distributed in the Member States, mainly among the 170 information centres. The HANDYNET database now contains around 48,000 items on technical aids and the organisations which manufacture and distribute them, along with 2000 illustrations of 1700 products.

The HANDYNET network has continued to hold assessment sessions in the various Member States. The draft HANDYNET evaluation report, which the Commission must submit to the Council and European Parliament in July 1994, was examined by the meeting of the HANDYNET technical co-ordination group and has now been adopted by the Commission for submission to Council and Parliament.

Evaluation of the HELIOS Programme

Many organisations from across Europe responded to a call for tender published in the Official Journal of the European Communities for a contractor to head an objective and independent evaluation of the HELIOS II Programme. The contract was eventually awarded to the Tavistock Institute in London, which heads a team from four countries including the European Centre for Work and Society (NL), Prisma (GR) and Nexus (IR). All four institutes have considerable experience in undertaking research in the social field and in evaluating major European programmes.

The evaluation to be undertaken by this team will address four key issues:

- In what ways and to what degree are disabled people and their families involved in the programme?
- By what means and to what extent has there been a transfer of effective and innovative practice and successful experiences at local, national and European levels?
- What is the value added to local activities of EC participation?
- To what extent has there been consultation and synergy with other relevant initiatives at local, national and European levels?

A number of principles will underpin the evaluation activities. One central principle is that disabled people are key 'stakeholders' in the evaluation of the programme, and for this reason a number of consultation mechanisms will be developed though which disabled people will be able to participate in the evaluation, set criteria by which the programme is evaluated, and provide their feedback on the impact of the progamme.

Another important principle is that the team's evaluation activities will build on and contribute to other local evaluations. The research team will therefore draw up an evaluation framework following initial consultations, and will also provide support for local evaluation activities via workshops. There will also be a number of other core activities, including a survey of participants in local activities, and case studies which will examine different aspects of the functioning of the programme.

PART III
An American Perspective

CHAPTER NINE

Vocational Rehabilitation Research in the United States of America

Frederick Menz

Introduction

The European Community is on the brink of its most exciting time; rehabilitation will be a significant part of that time.

This chapter is intended to convey a sense of how rehabilitation research endeavours in the United States come about, the scope of vocational rehabilitation research, and what my research group at the University of Wisconsin-Stout has been accomplishing over the past four of the 19 years we have maintained a national research centre in vocational rehabilitation. You will, perhaps, notice certain areas that may be of common interest or promise to the efforts within your own organizations. Finally, I will share my thoughts about what I feel are the most significant issues which vocational rehabilitation research must address.

The American Rehabilitation Research Scene

Let us begin by considering how rehabilitation research develops in the United States (*see* Figure 9.1). First and foremost, vocational rehabilitation research is a federal enterprise, supported through funds appropriated annually by the US Congress and, occasionally, other units of government, various professional organizations, the private sector, and charitable foundations. While research in medical rehabilitation (including applied and basic science related to physical restoration) receives significant funds through the private sector (e.g., pharmacological, technology companies), in addition to federal funds, that is not the case when it comes to vocational rehabilitation research. Across all agencies, the federal investment is probably no more than $100 to $200 million per year, with at least $50 million coming through one federal agency, the National Institute on Disability and Rehabilitation Research. Only a few million of the remaining dollars for rehabilitation research come from non-federal sources. However, more and more federal programmes are becoming concerned about vocational issues since people are surviving catastrophic injury for longer periods of time, disability claims and medical costs have skyrocketed, and people in those agencies have come to recognize that rehabilitation principles and technology apply to the problems disability creates for those agencies.

92 / VOCATIONAL REHABILITATION AND EUROPE

Second, vocational rehabilitation research is priority-based. That is, research does not 'mushroom' up through professions and disciplines with long traditions and commitments to inquiry and the development of 'scientific knowledge'. Rather, it comes about because of expressed national imperatives with significant political support. We in vocational rehabilitation remain a fairly practical lot.

```
                    Rehabilitation Act of 1973
                              │
                    U.S. Department of Education
                              │
                    Office of Special Education
                    and Rehabilitation Services
        ┌─────────────────────┼─────────────────────┐
  Rehabilitation         National Institute         Office of
    Services              on Disability and      Special Education
  Administration       Rehabilitation Research      Services
                              │
   ┌──────────┬───────────────┼───────────────┬──────────┐
 Research   Demonstration    Field         Fellowships  Special
and Training  Projects     Initiated                  Initiatives
  Center                   Research
```

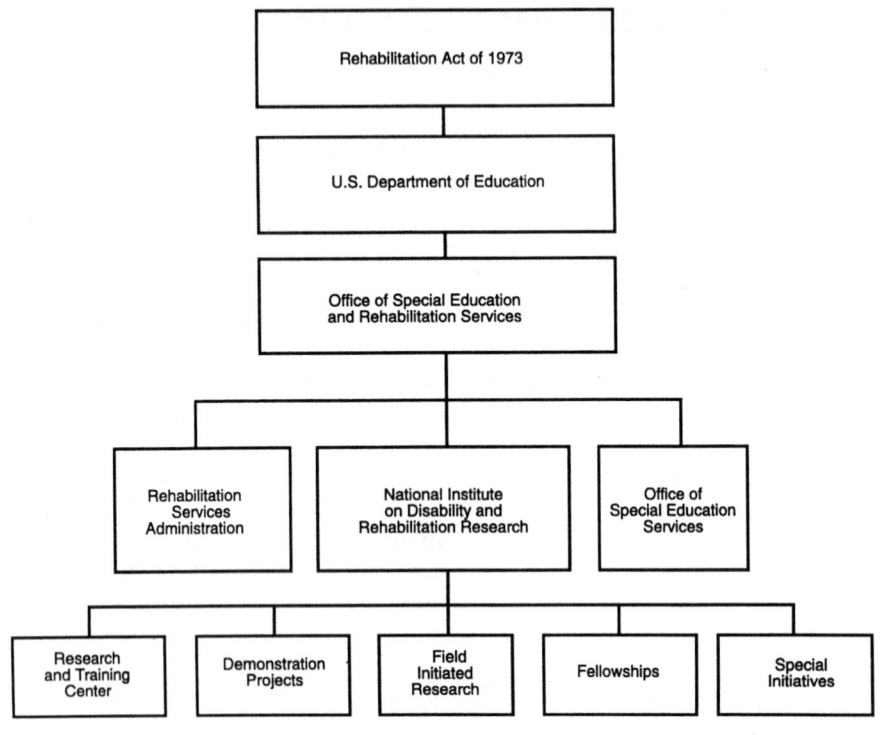

Figure 9.1. Formulation and Conduct of Vocational Rehabilitation Research in the United States

Political Advocacy in Formulation of Federal Programmes and Priorities

Consumers
Beneficiaries
Professionals
Providers
Governmental units
Associations
Universities
Private Sectors
Researchers
Economics
Geopolitical events

Figure 9.2. Political Advocacy

Third, this research is inextricably tied to the national effort to provide rehabilitation services and special education services to adults and children. Because it is tied to service, its scope and authority are prescribed under the same federal legislation that directs and funds vocational and other rehabilitation services needed by people with severe disabilities. Research is not intended to be a separate and distinct function. Rather, like the training of rehabilitation professionals, it is conceived as a means to promote the delivery of effective, quality services to meet the needs of Americans with severe disabilities.

It is the nature of American government that the legislation which provides its authority comes about as a result of political advocacy (Figure 9.2 depicts the constituencies involved in advocacy in the United States). This advocacy not only affects the substance of the initial legislation with creates a national programme. Among the other events and mechanisms it influences are:

- the regulations that translate legislative authority into programmes
- the levels to which the US Congress annually appropriates funds for rehabilitation services *and* research
- the leadership appointed to provide direction to the programme
- the selection and awards process
- the implementation and adoption of research practices
- the amendments introduced in other related legislation
- because most federal legislation for social programmes is time-limited, how dramatically that legislation is periodically reshaped.

The importance of political advocacy throughout America's social history has always been significant:

- from the writing of the US Constitution
- through the nation's change from a confederation of states to a federal form of government comprised of an executive, represented legislative, and judicial branches
- to the economic and military actions promoted through law and international policy
- to the formulation of interleaved departments in the federal government to provide for the commercial, defence, transportation, education, health, social service, and welfare needs of the country
- to the formation of a strong federal presence between the 1930s and 1960s in health, welfare, education, and social arenas; and
- to the decentralization of government and government sponsored programmes we have seen in the United States in the last two decades.

That political advocacy plays a significant role in forming and guiding social programmes has not changed in the present. Rather, it is where such advocacy now originates and the consequences such changes in advocacy's locus have gradually had on the foundations of rehabilitation programmes and rehabilitation research which are now most telling.

Origins of the Rehabilitation Programme

The national rehabilitation programme in the United States came about to meet needs of returning veterans who were seriously disabled by the Second World War. The focus of the programme was on veterans who had suffered significant physical disabilities and was designed to respond to needs arising from their physical disabilities. It stressed restoration and included a significant involvement of the technology of prosthetics. Responsibility for the rehabilitation programme split as the economic needs of these persons became increasingly apparent, in conjunction with their medical problems. The vocational needs of this group also required significant attention. Responsibility for rehabilitation was split between the medical (and the veterans' programmes) and other agencies involved in employment and public welfare for persons unable to take care of their own needs. Direction for rehabilitation, though, remained under a medical model.

In the late 1940s and the 1950s, the programme expanded to include non-veterans as 'clients' and to allow for other life-limiting and life-threatening disabilities as appropriate for services (e.g. neurological, physical, systemic) and industrially injured persons. Simultaneously, we began to see the emergence of a federal-state rehabilitation programme, the introduction of eligibility requirements, and much clearer references to a 'national programme' captured in federal legislation. The driving focus in the programme at this time was on 'restoring and returning' the individual to gainful employment. The population continued to be adults, particularly adults with prior employment histories.

Yankee ingenuity and success in industrial production were paralleled in the national thinking about 'a system of rehabilitation', complete with eligibility requirements and a status approach to rehabilitation. The system was modeled in part after the medical model (diagnose, repair, rehabilitate) and in part after the industrial model (design, engineer, sequence, produce adapted persons). This national system of rehabilitation came to be largely divided into four parts:

- a national agency with responsibilities for establishing regulations for a national rehabilitation programme; for providing basic funding for rehabilitation services, research, professional training, and co-ordination; and for linking relevant resources to achieve the Congressional intents
- a state programme responsible for identifying, counselling, and co-ordinating rehabilitation for persons with eligible disabilities
- a medical provider sector with responsibility for identifying extent of disability and basic needs of individuals who were severely affected enough to be eligible for the state rehabilitation programmes
- a vocational provider sector with dual responsibilities for assessment, training, and temporary employment for persons with 'fixable' disabilities and for long-term employment (or day care) of persons with 'intractable' disabilities.

The federal government, during this period, provided strong programme direction under the Department of Health, Education, and Welfare, backed up by hard-fought-for funds for the rehabilitation programme (including research) from the US Congress. Individuals with significant influence in Washington made dramatic impacts in the shaping of the programmes (e.g., Mary Switzer) and the programme shifted from its focus on medical restoration and came to be classified as a vocational rehabilitation programme. The state part secured its place in state governments (e.g., in education, labour); established policy to control who would be eligible to receive services; invested in processes to identify what was required to rehabilitate the client and what would be allowable under this eligibility programme. The rehabilitation professions also had their fledgling beginnings in this period; most notably rehabilitation counselling and rehabilitation medicine.

A medical diagnosis continued to underlie eligibility for the programme and in many respects continued to determine the course of rehabilitation for the 'target populations' served by the programme. Cause or origin of disability (e.g., war injuries) diminished as a concern under the evolving programme and the range of populations considered eligible for it expanded throughout the 1960s and 1970s. Populations variously considered eligible for the programme included the developmentally disabled, alcoholics, public offenders, culturally distinct (e.g., inner-city blacks, reluctant learners), mentally ill, children, school-age youth, and those affected by cardiovascular diseases. The language of disability emphasized 'groups of individuals' who were similarly characterized by disease or origin of disability.

As significantly increased federal resources were made available during this era of the Great Society, the Department of Education, the developmental disabilities administration, the Civil Rights Administration, and alcoholism institutes were created to right inequities and injustices. The rehabilitation programme shifted to where its forte was most prominent: vocational rehabilitation. Severity of disability and specific eligibility tests became priorities with passage of the 1973 Rehabilitation Act.

It is in this period of history that we find that vocational rehabilitation facilities, sheltered workshops, and day activity centres came into their own. Significant infusions of federal dollars were provided for their construction, state-federal resources were earmarked for their utilization, business and charitable involvement in their sponsorship came to be considered good social and community responsibility, and the need for trained and qualified rehabilitation professions was commonly promoted by government, providers, and advocates. We see, at this juncture, the specific rehabilitation professions identified in rehabilitation legislations and federal dollars directed toward both their pre-professional (i.e., for faculty and student stipends for degree programmes) and in-service training (i.e., funding for training individuals already working in specified rehabilitation roles).

Emergence of Collective Advocacy

With the 1986 Amendments to the Rehabilitation Act, we again saw changes of considerable importance to the rehabilitation programme arising from changes in our social values and the impact of political advocacy. These became presentiments of how changes would be brought about through advocacy. The source of advocacy efforts began to shift importance from single figures (e.g., Mary Switzer), who wielded substantial power to influence Congress and federal agencies, to collective power wielded through the hands of groups of individuals. This 'collective' advocacy was built upon the power realized through the Civil Rights Movement and it began to be wielded with greater importance in shaping the broad national goals for rehabilitation:

- 'vocational rehabilitation' was largely replaced in the language of the Act with 'rehabilitation'
- independent living was identified as a distinct service option for people without immediate vocational goals
- supported employment was identified as a distinct programme and outcome for the most severely disabled individuals
- American Indians and other underserved populations were identified as target populations for the federal-state rehabilitation programme; and
- requirements for need-based programming were introduced:
  - a formal state plan must be followed and based on the assessed needs of persons in the state with disabilities
  - eligibility must be based on expressed needs among severely disabled persons
  - an individualized rehabilitation plan must be developed based on individual needs, and
  - the state programme must be evaluated based on the extent to which it meets needs of persons with severe disabilities.

These changes irremediably set the basis for our present goal to put greatest control over the individual's rehabilitation programme in the hands of consumers of rehabilitation services.

Throughout the national-federal levels of government, the influences of successive Republican Administrations in the White House began to play out. Economic policy shifted from significant support for social programmes to the creation of capital, industry, and employment. Public policy, as it reflects social policy, shifted from strong federal control over programmes to increased expectations of state and local governments and of individual-private initiatives to solve social problems. Deregulation of federally created social, economic, welfare, and health programmes took place. Appropriation levels authorized by the Congress were reduced and, when allowable, the authority and funds for these programmes were transferred downward through very broadly defined initiatives and social philosophies (e.g., supported employment). Finally, concerns over an escalating national deficit began to be reflected in the passage of more restricted budgets, in increasingly micro-level legislation, and by the oversight studies conducted through the Office of Management and Budgets and by Congress. The accountants (called 'bean counters' by some) took over government planning.

Federal agencies were stripped of their planning, monitoring, and compliance powers as programme authority was shifted to the state, local, and private sectors. Efforts to consolidate planning of the rehabilitation programme at the federal level collapsed as control over its priorities and delivery changed hands. Democratization-decentralization challenged the basic tenets of a cohesive national policy and an integrated nationally supported coalition of rehabilitation programmes and resources. Prevailing political attitudes predicted the need for 'safety nets' as the Administration moved to a 'neo-federalism' and a restricted view of government's social responsibility: a responsibility for meeting needs of only those persons unable to assure their own safety and well-being; that is, the indigent poor, the most severely disabled, and...the failed corporation.

Measures of the quality of programmes were increasingly based on the 'dollars of similar benefits' which the 'invested' federal dollar leveraged through state, local, and private matching. Private contributions to charities (including to rehabilitation) and private sector commitments to employment of people with disabilities declined as corporate tax incentives disappeared and as the nation's industrial base began to shift from a hard industry base to an economy linked to technology, information, and personal services. Public dollars for rehabilitation shrank, shifted to other programmes, and moved downward to government units with goals based on regional priorities, of which rehabilitation would be one of many competing concerns (e.g., crime, unemployment, urban decay, public transportation).

However, with very real needs still present, a better informed electorate in place, a growing dissatisfaction with the difference between promise and delivery in government-sponsored programmes, and an apparent loss of support for rehabilitation efforts, collective advocacy obtained a major injection of enthusiasm and support. Public activism and organized advocacy came of age. This collective advocacy spawned unique alliances between similarly concerned proponents of causes and at the same time seriously separated historically invested constituencies into separate camps (e.g., bureaucrats, providers, the professions). Collective advocacy took to shaping social and political attitudes around issues critical to groups of individuals affected by similar disabilities (e.g., parents of children and adults with developmental disabilities). Specific philosophies of quality of life and approaches to solving problems of disabilities became aggressively advocated and pursued as the 'right alternatives'. That is, the socially responsible processes.

The combined force of this activism, actually, brought about passage of the Americans with Disabilities Act of 1990. The diverse and many voices of such activism can also be expected to alter significantly the substance of Rehabilitation Act. It is very likely that such a shift will transfer increased control over the programme in the hands of consumers; the person directly affected by disability. Demands for rehabilitation that meets 'my needs' will not only be heard, but will likely become integral to the design of the entire rehabilitation enterprise in the United States.

The monumentally important Americans with Disabilities Act needs a vehicle through which its intended impacts on access to employment, housing, transportation, and public accommodations can be realized. The successful application of political advocacy which brought about passage of that Act demonstrated, for collective advocacy, a strength that will neither be ignored nor diminished. Collective advocacy's enthusiasm will be challenging all of the principles, processes, and priorities of rehabilitation in the United States; including those for service and for research, even though priorities for research may seem to be a long way down on advocacy's list. Realities of the present tell us that the endeavours, designs, and guidance for rehabilitation in the United States will be:

- greatly influenced by continuing collective political advocacy
- increasingly focused on the needs of individuals with severe disabilities
- more likely to be conceived and guided by democratic principles
- more costly and difficult to provide; and
- more concerned about value added for dollar invested.

Subsequent reauthorizations of the Rehabilitation Act and the instituting of the Americans with Disabilities Act will be affected by these constraints. Consumer choice, value for dollar invested, and benefits to individuals with profound disabilities will more and more shape rehabilitation delivery, including its historic hand maiden, vocational rehabilitation research.

National Institute on Disability and Rehabilitation Research

Throughout the 1970s and early 1980s, vocational rehabilitation cherished its heyday of federal support because of the evident return on investment that could be traced to the rehabilitation of people with disabilities: up to $30 in recovered taxes on earnings for every federal and state dollar invested in a successful rehabilitation. No other social programme could evidence such benefits to the nation's economy. Rehabilitation and special education programmes were moved from 'Welfare' to the Department of Education. The National Institute on Disability and Rehabilitation Research (though variously named during this period) was established as a functional unit in the Office of Special Education and Rehabilitation Services within the Department of Education. (Figure 9.3 shows the Institute's relationship to rehabilitation under the Department of Education.)

At the same time, rehabilitation medicine came to be the fastest growing medical discipline and the vocational rehabilitation professions and programmes (counselling, evaluation, adjustment, placement) came into their greatest acceptance. Accreditation efforts for rehabilitation service providers were established by the Commission on Accreditation of Rehabilitation Facilities. Certification of qualified rehabilitation professionals was begun for the professions (i.e., rehabilitation counselling, then vocational evaluation). Resources to support the programmes and to provide employment for disabled Americans came about at this same time (e.g., National Industries for the Severely Handicapped, set-aside programmes for purchase of products and services from rehabilitation facilities by federal and state agencies). The balance of dollars between vocational-medical rehabilitation began its shift toward non-medical services, to personnel development, and to research and development.

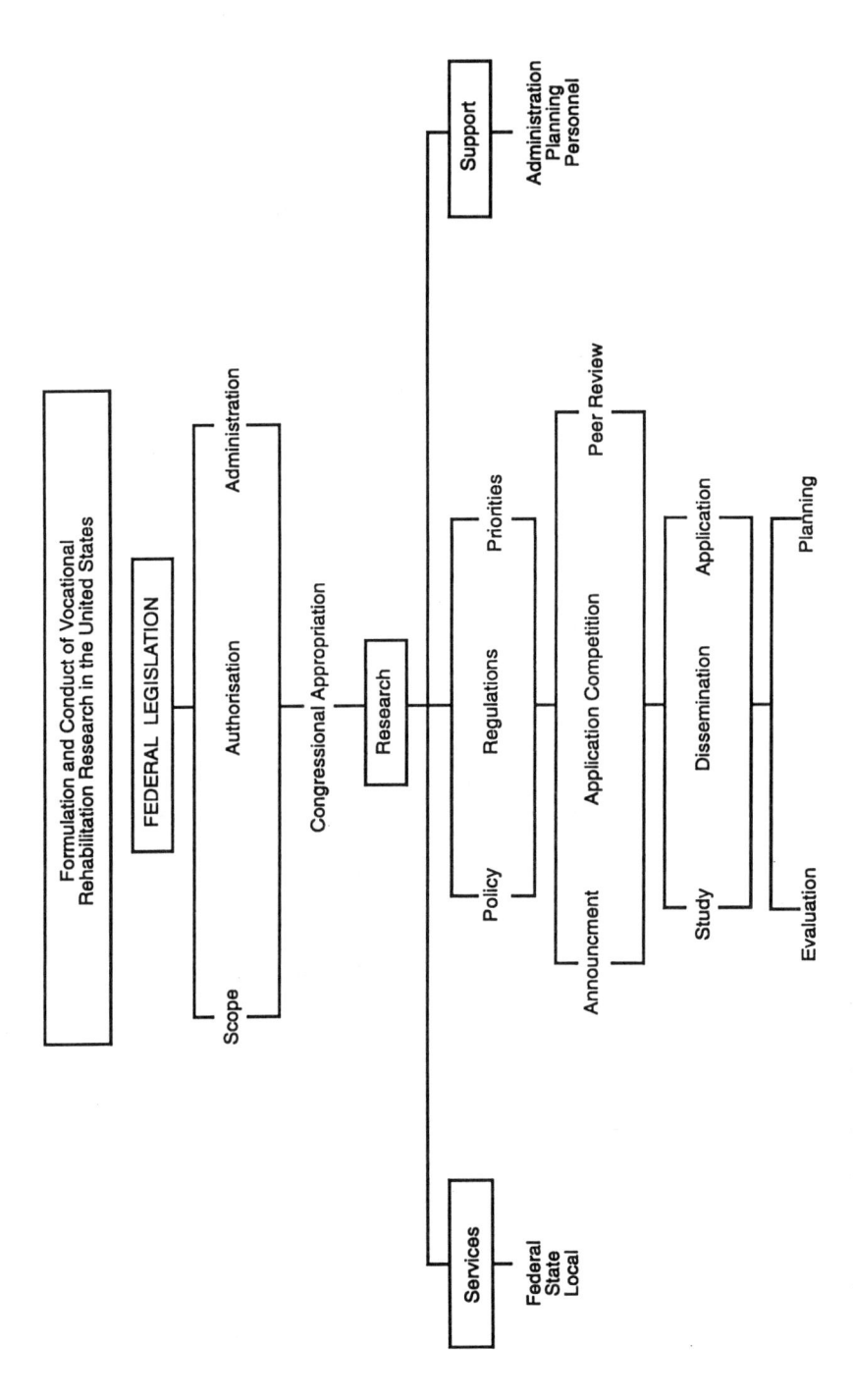

Figure 9.3. The Institute's Relationship to Rehabilitation and Special Education

Participatory Action Research

A national rehabilitation research policy is beginning to emerge, which in many respects is more in keeping with shifts in political advocacy than the national-state rehabilitation programme as a whole. The Director of the National Institute on Disability and Rehabilitation Research has gone on public record to offer alternatives to the present manner in which research is wed with rehabilitation practice.

> In traditional approaches to disability and rehabilitation research, the role of the person with a disability is that of a subject, an object to be investigated. The problem investigated is usually defined as a physical, sensory, communication, cognitive, or mental impairment, employability, functional limitations, or lack of motivation and cooperation of the person with the disability. The locus of the research problem is in the individual with the disability. The research strategy is usually determined by the researcher. The strategy is often an intervention designed by the rehabilitation professional or researcher addressing the problem identified by the researcher... The researcher is in control of the research design from the formulation of the research question to the outcomes promoted to the dissemination of the knowledge produced and the products shared. (Graves 1991, pp.16–17)

Although the data in Figure 9.4 are hypothetical, the figure conveys the essence of the problem. Rehabilitation research produces minimal new practices or

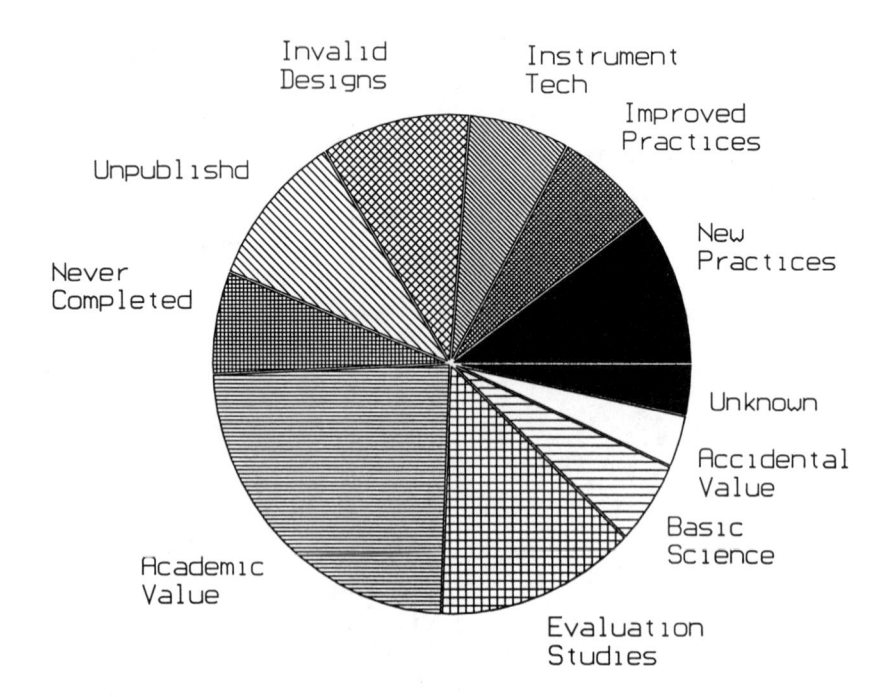

Figure 9.4. Utility of Rehabilitation Research (Hypothetical)

solutions to current practices problems because consumers (i.e., people with disabilities) are not integral to the research effort. Graves' evaluation of rehabilitation research concludes that the problem, and solutions, are too often in the wrong hands. The processes are too non-interactive and not involving enough of the consumer and other constituencies that are to be affected by the consequences of the research or involving enough of those responsible for carrying out a practice derived from research. Participatory Action Research (PAR) causes inclusion and involvement of the individuals of interest, not as objects of inquiry, but as full participants in all stages of the research endeavour: from problem formulation through design and into application. Graves states that the National Institute

> ...will encourage the use of PAR to promote better science. PAR is neither a quantitative nor a qualitative approach to disability and rehabilitation research. Rather PAR is a paradigm that maximizes involvement and participation of the consumer of the research in the research policies and outcome – be that consumer a person with a disability, a parent, spouse, or sibling of a person with a disability, or a rehabilitation services provider...PAR is a paradigm...that will enhance the quality, rigour, and usefulness of the research endeavour, and it will strengthen the partnership between the disability and research community and research consumers. (Graves 1991, pp.25–26)

This strong sentiment may radically reshape how the ends towards which America's involvement in rehabilitation research and development will work. Again, though the data are hypothetical, Figure 9.5 conveys the essence of how consumers (i.e., people with disabilities) might benefit through a revitalization of America's efforts in rehabilitation research.

In a federal environment with very limited resources for research, dollars retained count triple. First, they are dollars not lost. Second, they are dollars that do not have to be negotiated out of some other agencie's budget. Third, they are dollars which escaped the 'primary fluff-cuts' which research and development funds so often experienced. Such retention of research dollars, though, requires political capital. Political capital today means that the dollars set aside for research must provide 'valued' benefits: research which provides improvements of apparent or immediate value and qualitative contributions to individual attainments are considered of greater importance. Research for science, for knowledge building, for capacity building, or of conceptual and individual interest to the researcher are of lesser value when such pay-offs are compared. Research for research alone cannot be justified under these conditions.

At this time, as Figure 9.5 suggests, the need is for significantly improved quality of rehabilitation practices and the claim is that America's vocational rehabilitation research does not have a sufficiently high yield in improved and new rehabilitation practices. The utility of rehabilitation research for rehabilitation practice must be dramatically increased. The time-gap between research and practice must be narrowed. This policy proposes an important refocus for federally sponsored research with regard to the way in which the identification, documentation, and determination of new and improved practices. The time-gap

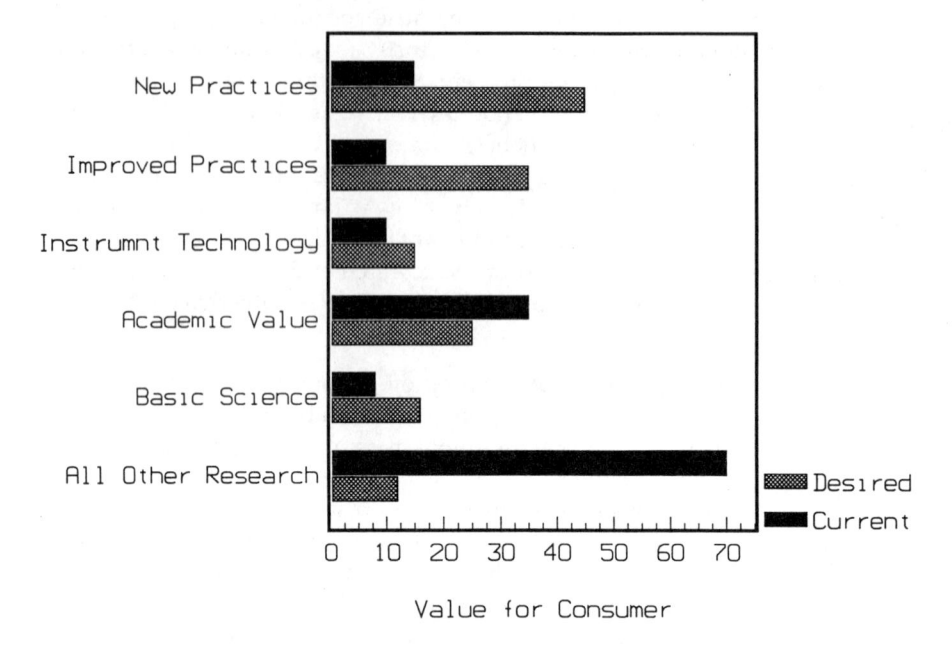

[Bar chart showing Desired vs Current Value for Consumer across categories: New Practices, Improved Practices, Instrumnt Technology, Academic Value, Basic Science, All Other Research]

Figure 9.5. Anticipated Impacts to be Achieved (Hypothetical)

between research and practice must be narrowed. The paradigm shift proposed by Dr Graves is in keeping with social attitudes and political advocacy which has shifted toward increased participation and direction by people with disabilities. Like the services to which rehabilitation research is considered wed, vocational rehabilitation research must make definite and meaningful impacts on solutions to problems resulting from disability and must be meaningful to people affected by disability within the United States. As the above figure suggests, participatory action research is geared to increasing the immediate benefits from research. It proposes a process which may increase sensitivity to the identification, improvement, and validation of the practices used with individuals affected by disabilities.

Under PAR, individuals with disabilities must be integrally involved in the design of rehabilitation processes if those processes are to work and be accepted, and can, therefore, influence the quality and meaningfulness (i.e., the internal validity) of such applied research. Research that does not respect such a point of view may not survive. As the figure suggests, the objective is to produce better science and better application: vocational rehabilitation research is linked to vocational rehabilitation delivery. Support for rehabilitation research will expand, as this position proposes, when that link is strengthened and the bond between the two result in a complementary marriage with progeny named 'quality', 'impact', and 'social value'.

What Kinds of Research are being Funded

Social goals underlie what research is funded, how well it is funded, and how sensitive researchers remain to the broader needs of the persons in the community of disability. This is not to detract, in any fashion, from how creatively, conscientiously, and rigorously rehabilitation research is conducted in the United States. What is promoted as public policy and agency regulations is not responded to in an autonomic fashion. Like their counterparts throughout Europe, researchers are still generally housed at institutions of higher learning, are trained to revile simplism and dogmatism, and have been acculturated to revere their individual pursuit of truth through the processes of research and intellectual inquiry. They are still as self-assured and as arrogant as you might expect from people with high intelligence, who are products of rigorous academic training, and who have to live up to the demanding expectations of their colleagues on a daily basis.

Social attitudes, translated into agency policy, guide and shape the research of those successful in achieving research awards from the agency. Such policy influences and also creates various options to help forge a more productive link between science and application. While an agency's policy does not enforce an adherence to one scientific process over another, it does challenge the community of scientists to consider both the urgency of the problems that need solutions and their peculiar capacities to assist more readily in resolving those problems. For some of our greatest rehabilitation problems, the rate of progress in science cannot be dramatically increased. For example, questions of the comparability and sustained benefits achieved by sheltered people moved from employment to supported employment cannot be answered through some experiment with carefully collected random samples, because present time is not sufficient to allow the assessment of those benefits; the programme is too new. For other of our great problems, science cannot arrive at the needed, precise answers demanded by individuals directly affected by a disability. For instance, how ageing, pre-existing conditions, and traumatic injury combine to affect the onset and course of dysfunction is now only beginning to be understood as more individuals have survived the acute stages and have progressed through rehabilitation.

Yet, as regards other problems, the challenge will not be to unearth reliable, new knowledge, but to reconsider and focus the expertise and technology of research to understanding and explicating what does and does not work. We may need more often to choose not to chase the 'elusive hypothesis' (keeping in mind that doing so is what we as researchers-in-the-guise-of-scientists do if we want to achieve image, publications, tenure, and promotions), but instead choose to work with real people in real settings to verify what it is reliably achieved with certain individuals and how those effects are achieved. Probably among the greatest challenges, to those of us who think of ourselves as scientists, will be responsibly to reconcile our professional needs to look into the unknown and pursue questions of interest to our own intellectual growth and, perhaps, a responsibility to join such curiosity to solving some of the broader social issues to which our skills may add the new critical value.

Rehabilitation Research and Training Centres

The National Institute on Disability and Rehabilitation Research is funded to the tune of about $50 million per year to support a network of Research and Training Centres, Rehabilitation Engineering Centres, demonstration projects, field-initiated research, research fellowships, and special initiatives. For instance, special initiatives have been funded by the Institute for dissemination of information about the Americans with Disabilities Act and for training employers and others in how to respond responsibly to the provisions of that Act. Figure 9.6 indicates the distribution of Centres across the United States.

These 40 Research and Training Centres are, in my estimation, the cornerstone of the national programme of research in that they are designed to bring critical resources to solving long-term issues in disability, are funded for several years, and are typically located at institutions where long-term support can ensure that their programmatic missions are accomplished in the general priority areas for which they are funded. The number of Centres varies, depending on changes in fundamental priorities, and has nearly doubled over the past 20 years. They provide the long-term ground both from which subsistence crops can be harvested and on which forests of hardwoods can be achieved to insure the nutrition, clean air, and water needed by people in our respective disciplines who attempt to serve, today and tomorrow, disability needs across the country.

In 1972 there were 22 Centres funded, most with physical medicine emphases, a few focused on specific disabilities, and three with vocational emphases. As Figure 9.6 attempts to show, there has been a significant shift in national priorities mirrored by the mission areas of these 40 Centres. Note the small number of Centres dealing with medical issues, keeping in mind that none of these are now funded to do 'basic science', but all are engaged in research relevant to vocational rehabilitation interventions. Note also the number of Centres with missions in 'employment-vocational'. Finally, note the significant number of Centres dealing with specific populations and the broad spectrum of options now allowable under the Rehabilitation Act: Native Americans, minorities, Pacific Islanders, children, ageing, independent living, community-integration, public policy.

Each of these research centres has dual functions in research (that has potential application for persons served through the state-federal rehabilitation system) and in training of professionals-practitioners in the outcomes and practices the research produces. Much of their training is applied in professional training programmes. In recent years, some of that training has been directed toward consumers, their families, and policy-makers. Much of the research is published through project reports and in the professional journals throughout the United States. There is no federal control over publications from these research centres. However, all publications and products are supposed to be provided to and made available through the National Rehabilitation Information Centre, at Washington, DC. Too much of the research, though, is only seen in annual reports to the National Institute, is reported in fugitive documents at the Centres, or is conveyed to limited audiences through presentations like the one from which this paper was prepared.

VOCATIONAL REHABILITATION RESEARCH IN THE USA / 105

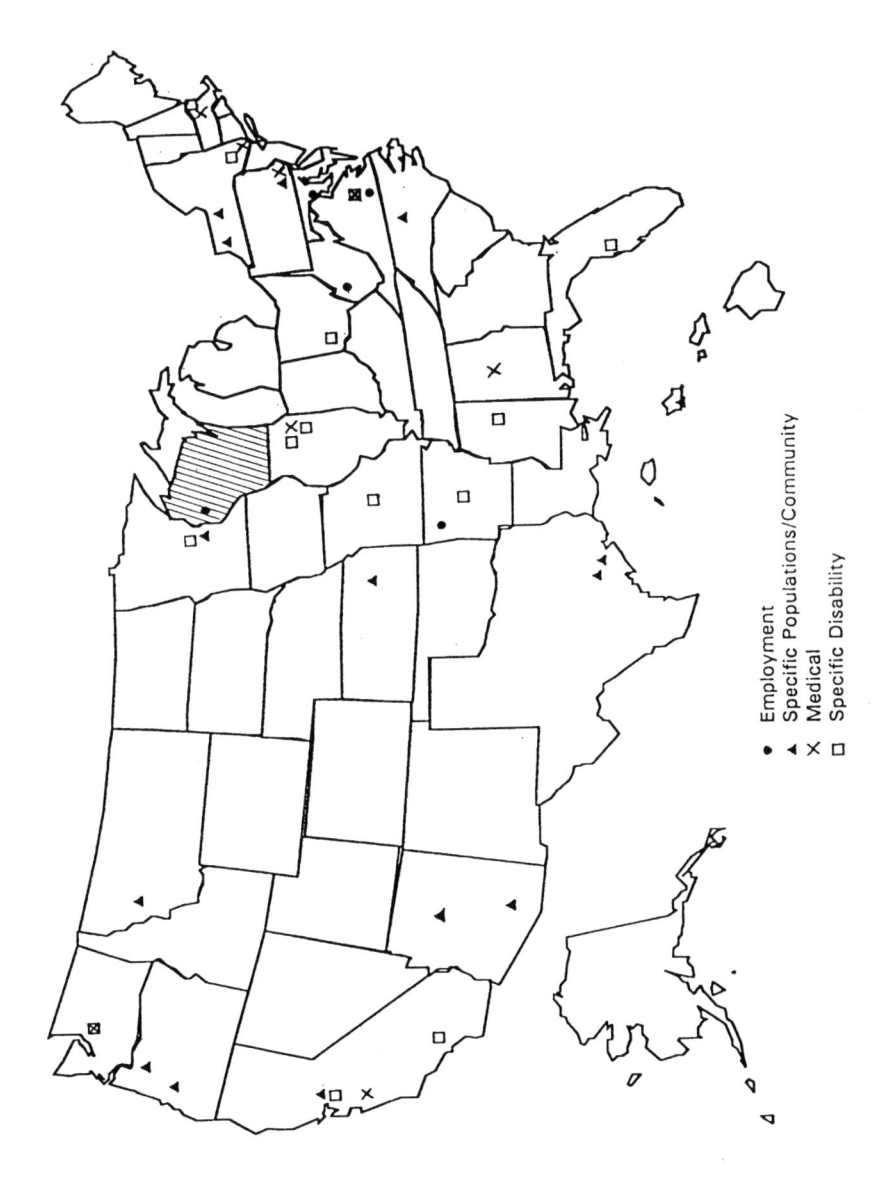

- • Employment
- ◂ Specific Populations/Community
- × Medical
- ☐ Specific Disability

Figure 9.6. Research Missions of the 40 Centres in 1991

Vocational Rehabilitation Research at the University of Wisconsin-Stout Research and Training Centre

Shading on the Figure 9.6 map outlines the state of Wisconsin where our research centre resides. The Research and Training Centre at the University of Wisconsin-Stout was first funded in 1972 to conduct research and training relevant to professionals working in rehabilitation facilities. While we are housed at a state university, the scope of our research programme is not guided by that institution. As we have already noted, the United States' state-federal programme includes a federal component, a state level system, and the private sector service resources. The state system guides an individual through a rehabilitation plan and uses its federal and state money to purchase necessary services from a disjointed community-local level collection of rehabilitation facilities which provide medical and vocational services.

Our Centre's Mission

Our research programme addresses issues of importance to the provision of services at this community level. Historically, it has concentrated on 'what can be provided to people with various disabilities *in* the facility'. These research issues were predicated upon a concern for how such services as vocational evaluation, work adjustment, placement, supported employment, and extended employment were provided through the vocational rehabilitation facility. Each five years new national priorities are identified and guide our research planning. Priorities change as needs for new information and guidance in the field have changed. At present, the Centre is concentrating on 'how the facility can move as much of its services into natural or community settings'.

Mission

Using the processes of research and development and the techniques of training, dissemination, and collaboration, assist rehabilitation facilities to adopt those new programme and practice options which a) increase the availability and efficiency of community-based employment programmes and b) enhance opportunities for individuals with disabilities to access, obtain, and maintain employment that affords them community integration and competitive benefits from their work.

Figure 9.7. Mission of UW-Stout's Research and Training Centre

The Centre's research activities are controlled by the research plan it submits to the National Institute as part of a competitive application process and the Centre's mission (presented in Figure 9.7). The plan changes as the research programme matures, but the mission remains constant. As that mission suggests, the research is geared toward community-based employment models and the systems necessary to maximize select consumer goals (i.e., employment, integration).

In this five-year cycle, the Centre is also attending to the unique needs of persons with traumatic brain injury or with severe psychiatric disabilities. Most projects we conduct are three- to five-year studies. Short-term research studies are entertained as appropriate to longer-term programmatic research goals, often conducted by staff in conjunction with graduate students and clinical colleagues around the country. Collectively, the projects are to have a strong applications component. Consumers and rehabilitation constituencies are consulted at critical stages of the research. A wide range of methods are used to acquire information, data, and understanding of the basic research and potential applications issues. Clinical, experimental, survey, and consensus methodologies are variously used. Qualitative and quantitative approaches are used in both field studies and with consumers, professionals, and national leaders and policy-makers.

Status of the Vocational Rehabilitation Facility

Quite simply put, our research is expected to help meet the needs rehabilitation facilities have for providing better quality rehabilitation services. There are somewhere around 7000 rehabilitation facilities spread throughout the United States providing vocational rehabilitation and other rehabilitation services; both facility-based and community-based. These facilities represent an economic factor of no small proportions in the American rehabilitation scene.

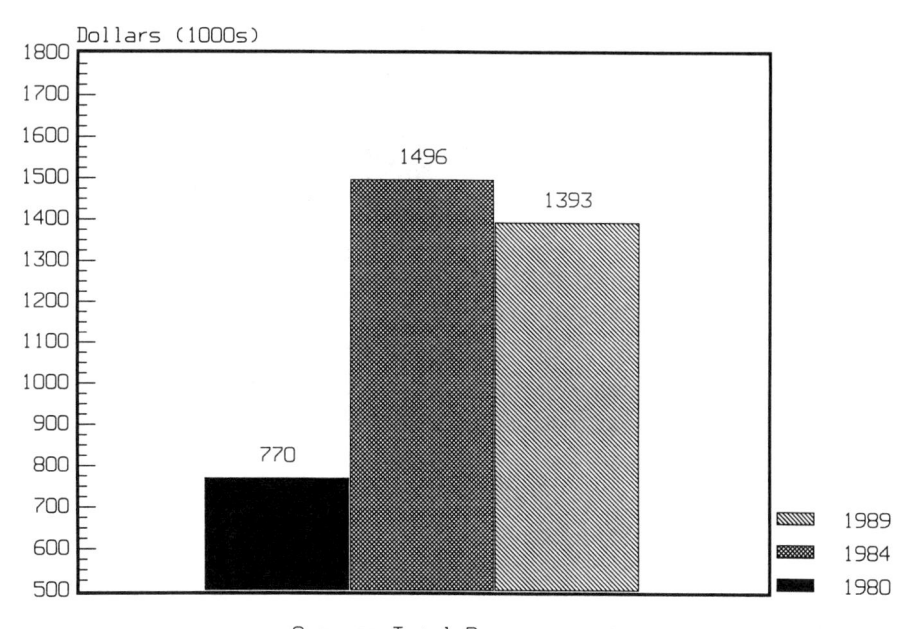

Figure 9.8. Changing Facility Economics

108 / VOCATIONAL REHABILITATION AND EUROPE

Projected out from the data in Figure 9.8, these facilities have combined revenues upwards of perhaps $9.8 billion dollars per year; roughly five times the $1.7 billion dollars the US Congress appropriates for the services portion of the basic states programme. As the state-level programmes do not spend more than 30 per cent of their service dollars in vocational rehabilitation facilities, it is clear that other sources than the vocational rehabilitation programme are relied upon to support the rehabilitation and employment programmes these facilities provide for their communities: non-fees sources of revenues account for 48 per cent of total revenues; fees from programmes for developmentally disabled and mental illness account for 46 per cent of their fee income; only 31 per cent of their fee income comes directly from the state vocational rehabilitation programme. Note that charitable contributions account for very small proportions of operating funds and that source has decreasing importance to sustaining the facility in American communities.

Severity of disability among persons served in vocational rehabilitation has increased and other organizations are increasingly serving the vocational needs of less severely affected individuals (see Figure 9.9).

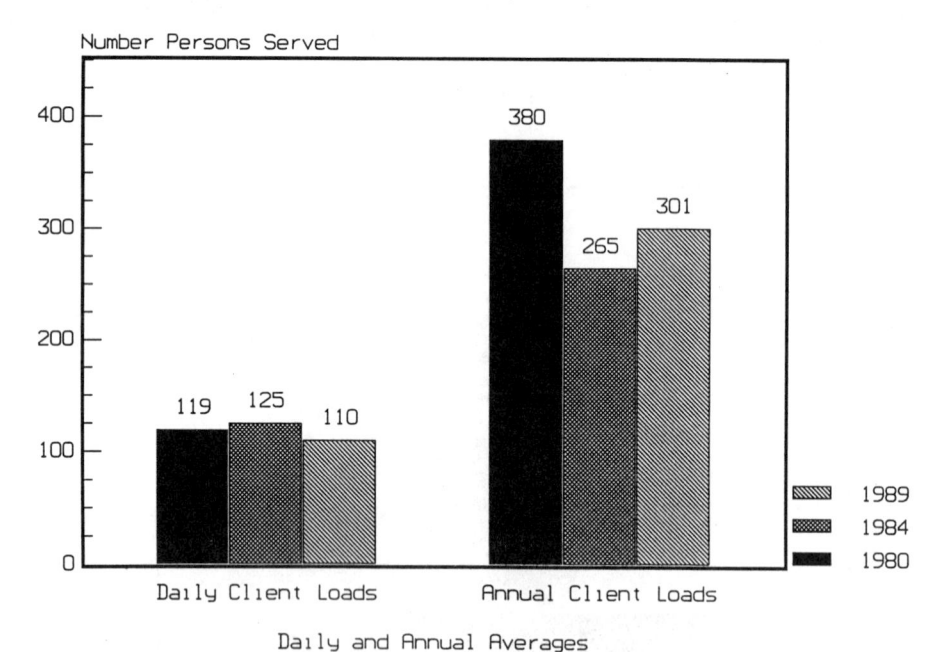

Figure 9.9. Changing Facility Size

Daily client loads and annual numbers of clients served in facilities have gradually declined. Yet upwards of two million individuals are provided services through facilities each year. Cognitively (55 per cent), psychiatrically (13 per cent), and multiply disabled (20 per cent) persons are comprising greater proportions of the daily and annual caseloads seen in rehabilitation facilities. While nearly 22 per cent of facility clients are now from minority populations, over 55 per cent have not graduated from high school (our 12th-year basic education degree). In keeping with general historic trends in vocational rehabilitation, only 8 per cent of individuals served in rehabilitation facilities have physical disabilities (as their primary disability), including persons with traumatic brain injury. Sixty per cent of people receiving services are in what should be their most productive working years (18–55 years), and 14 per cent are in their late careers (55–65 years).

Roughly one-half of the clients served in facilities receive employment or employment experience employment programmes and, generally, about 60 per cent of their training will be facility-based. In 1989, a person entering a facility had a one-in-four that one or more of their services would be provided in community-based settings, and that ratio was more favourable if skills training was involved. As Figure 9.10 depicts, employment provided through facilities was slightly better than half-time (we use a 40-hour work week as a reference point). Wages are paid based on the productivity of the individual relative to prevailing industrial or community standards for comparable jobs and, therefore, hourly earnings are well below minimum wage (for 1989, this was under $4.25 per hour). This was roughly the status of rehabilitation facilities as we began the current cycle of the Centre's vocational rehabilitation research programme.

Research and Development in Traumatic Brain Injury Models

The research conducted at the Centre can be divided into two parts: models development and studies of individual special needs which contribute to suc-

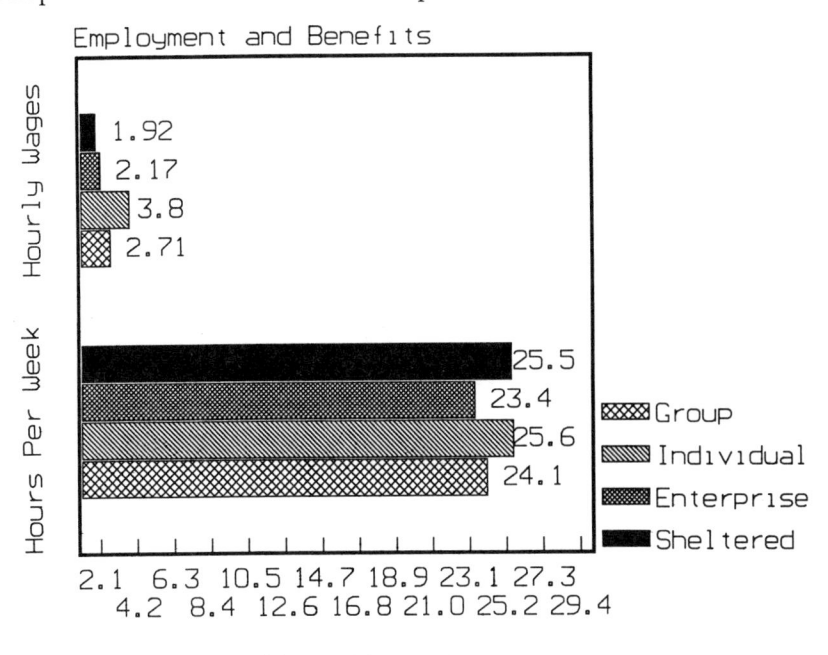

Figure 9.10. Earnings in Employment

cessful model development. This division is purely for intellectual convenience, however, in that we find ourselves continually crossing back and forth between issues of individual needs and getting new materials with which to construct our models. Let me begin to talk about this research with an examination of a popular alternative to community-based services: supported employment. This is research by my colleague, Dale Thomas, and it raises considerable questions about that model's efficacy because the demonstration study not only tested a model in rural America, it also attempted to identify broad practical and systemic issues in programming with persons with traumatic brain injury.

Project HIRe (Head Injury Re-entry) attempted to apply a supported employment model with strong assessment (vocational/neurological), placement, and assistive supports (on and off the job) to persons living in two rural communities, Menomonie in Wisconsin and Rochester in Minnesota, plus an initial developmental site at the University. The critical elements of the model are shown in Figure 9.11. Neither location had an extensive population base; both areas had a very small number of key employers and many smaller employers; and in both locations individuals in the programme were very severely affected and tended to reside outside the 'town' setting.

Assessment and Planning Stage

Referral and Intake
Planning the Evaluations
Vocational Assessment
Neuropsychological Evaluation
Planning Employment, Training, and Supports

Community-Based Employment and Training Stage

Alternative Paths
Placement and Replacement
Job Skills Training and Monitoring
Planning for Community and Job Supports
Movement Between Jobs
Preparing for Transfer

Maintenance Stage

Transfer to Long-Term Coaching
Insuring Long-Term Supports are in Place
Financial Supports
Employment Supports
Other Support Needs to Consider
Maintaining Linkages

Figure 9.11 The HIRe Model Stages and Steps

As the model began to be developed, we thought we would be able to serve 30 or more individuals at each site. We learned our first lesson almost from the onset: disability density is much less in rural areas; resource needs are much greater than anticipated; resource availability is much more dispersed; and getting long-term funding for supports was significantly more difficult in these less densely populated counties.

We were ultimately able to deal with the demands placed on our project resources as we reduced the number of persons we would serve. But, as Figure 9.12 suggests, the overall demands for *on- and off-job* support was considerably more than might have been predicted. In Figure 9.12, these averages are based across 74 weeks when individuals were working.

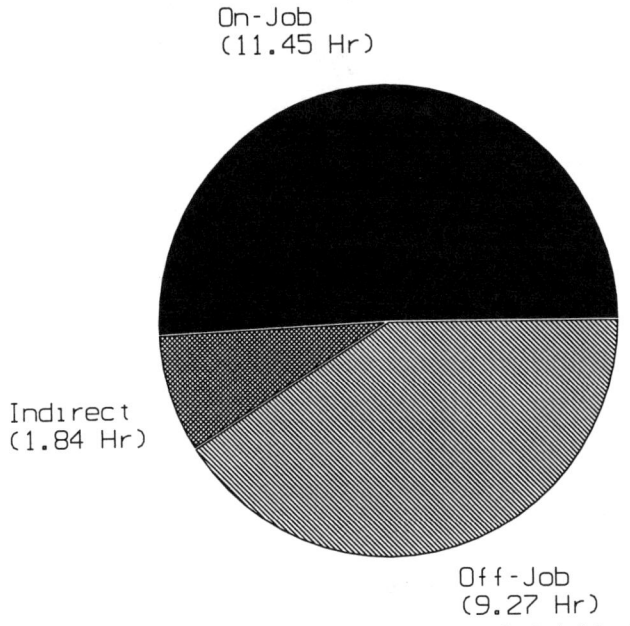

Figure 9.12. Distribution of 17.23 Hours of Support During Work Week (N = 14)

There were two findings we found especially surprising. Given the severity of disability, we were not surprised by the level of on-the-job support they required, nor that it was so high across the employment period. What was unexpected was the amount of off-the-job support that was needed.

As Figure 9.13 shows, such support did not deal with housing (they were living with families or in established congregate housing), but with their personal finances, transportation, recreation, and getting to and from essential services. These needs did not occur at work; but were important to being able to maintain employment.

The second finding we were surprised by was the extent to which support was required throughout their employment and the variability of support requirements between individuals. Figures 14, 15, 16, and 17 graphically display how intense support was across the weeks of employment and how the needs

112 / VOCATIONAL REHABILITATION AND EUROPE

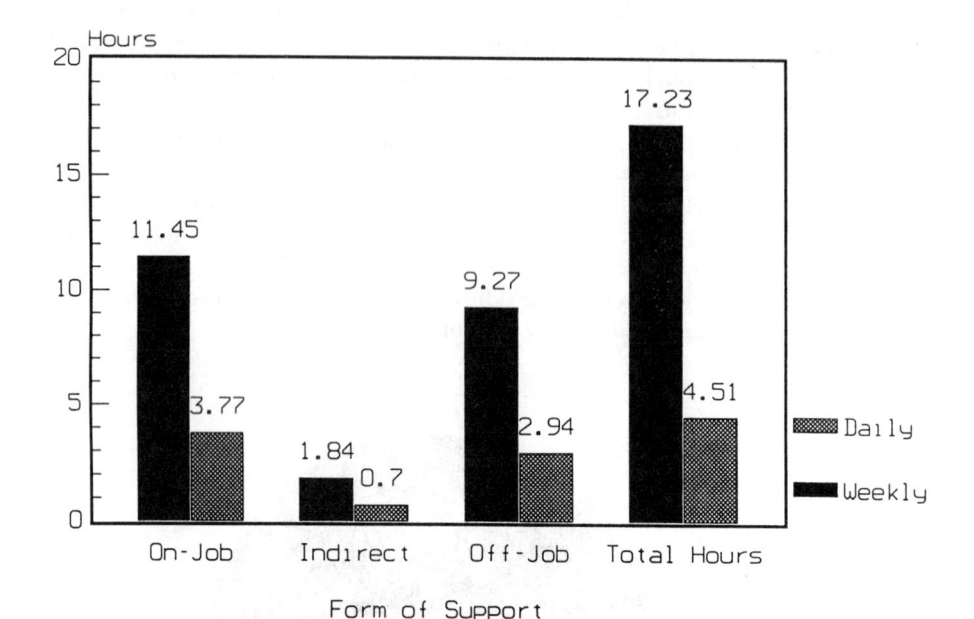

Figure 9.13. Distribution of Supports Provided to 14 Persons in Community-Based Employment

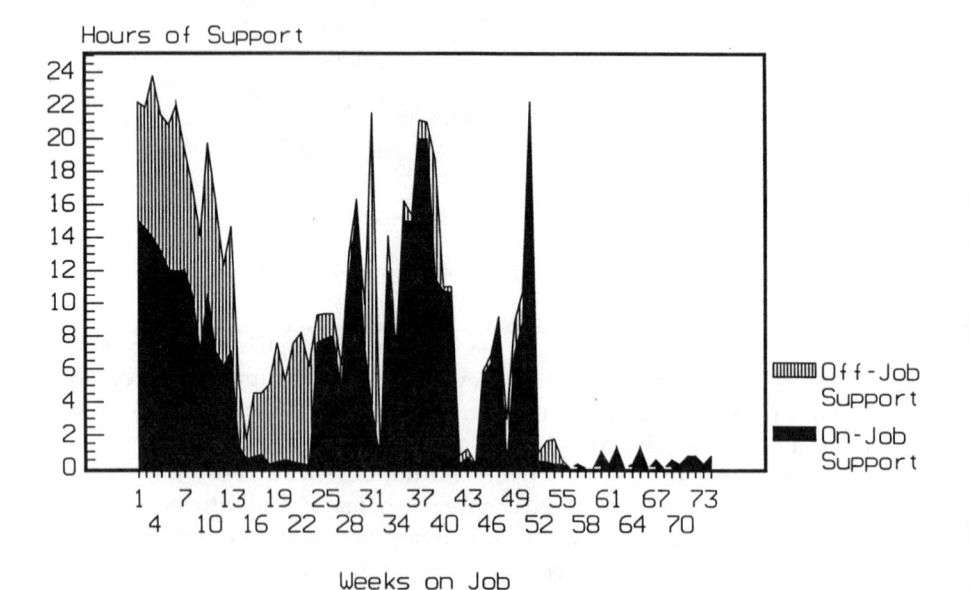

Figure 9.14. Changes in On- and Off-Job Support Needed by Persons With Traumatic Brain Injury in Community-Based Employment

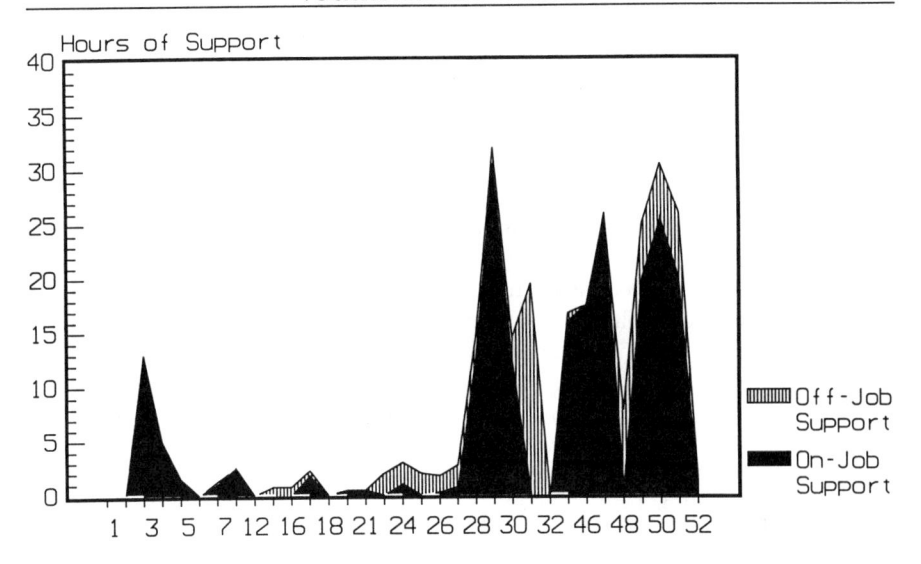

Figure 9.15. On-Off Job Support for Ss 127 During 52 Weeks of Employment

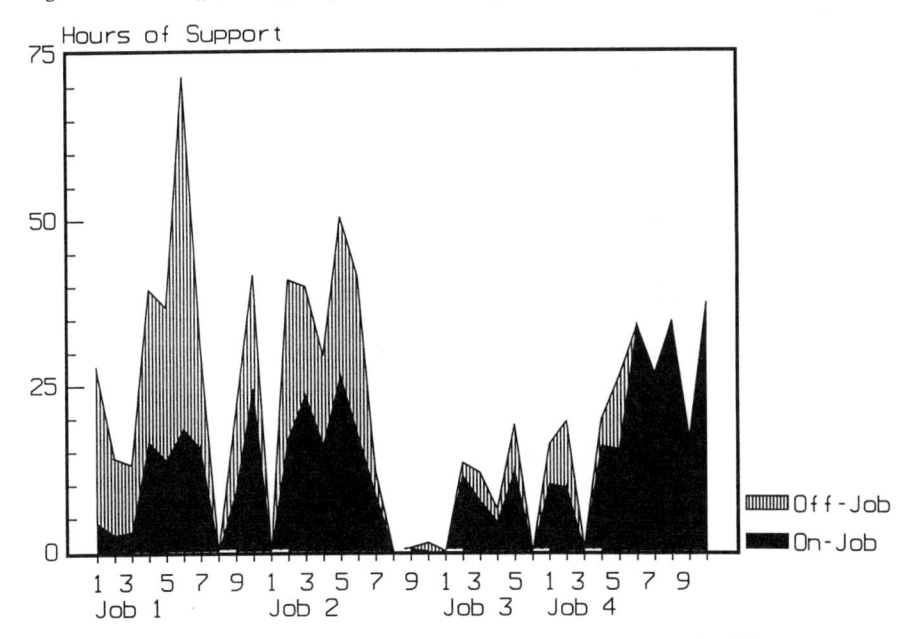

Figure 9.16. On- and Off-Job Supports for Ss 118 During Four Community Jobs

114 / VOCATIONAL REHABILITATION AND EUROPE

varied among individuals. Figure 14 shows the overall pattern of on-off job support for all 14 subjects over the 74 weeks. The next three figures show these patterns for an individual who maintained a job for 52 weeks and then patterns for two individuals who held multiple jobs. These later figures dramatically demonstrate the point about individual variability.

Not only were the demands on rural resources much more acute than expected, the substance of supports was quite different from that originally found by Paul Wehman and his colleagues in supported employment with developmentally disabled individuals. The predicted method of intensive on-the-job training and support, followed by relatively low levels of maintenance support, did not consistently occur among these traumatically brain-injured individuals. Instead, different patterns of on-/off-job interventions were found between individuals and were linked to changes in employment and changes occurring on the job.

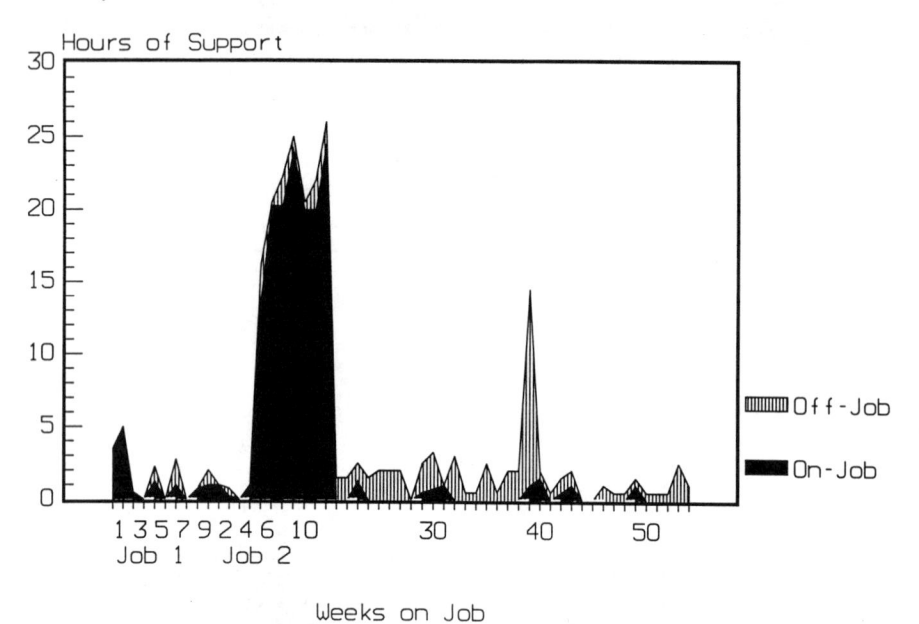

Figure 9.17. Subject 25 On- and Off-Job Supports on Two Community Jobs

As Figure 9.18 indicates, these individuals required 11.5 hours of on-job support, 9.3 hours of off-job support, and 1.8 hours of indirect support for every 21 hours a week they worked. Assuming for the moment that we were to pay a job coach $8.00 per hour, the average cost per week for support will run at least $168 against earnings from work of about $73. In their last job under HIRe, 10 of the 17 were earning above minimum wage and two returned to non-supported competitive employment.

This model development experience has provided a considerable lesson as displayed on Figure 9.19. Supported employment can work with these individuals, but it does cost and requires concentration with especially high qualities.

Number of Workers	17
Overall Employment Pattern and Benefits	
Average number of jobs	2
Average weeks of support	17.6
Average hours support per week	17.2
On-job	11.5
Off-job	9.3
Indirect	1.8
Average hourly rate	3.05
Per cent possible weeks worked	89.9
Employment Benefits Last Job	
Average hourly rate	3.45
Average hours per week	21
Average weeks worked with supports	17
Persons referred to competitive employment	2
Number workers earning above minimum wage	10
Number at or below minimum wage	7

Figure 9.18. Employment Benefits Achieved at HIRe Replication Sites

Staffing for the model
  Employment training specialist as job coach
  Maintenance job coach
  Clinical team approach to rehabilitation
  Staff development and preparation

Desirable features of assessment
  Coordinated neuropsychological and vocational assessments
  Neuropsychological instrumentation
  Critical focus on vocational goals

Alternate contexts for training and assessment
  Psychometrics and work samples
  Situation assessments
  Monitored job trails
  Protected work sites
  Community-based work sites

Community advisory committee

Eligibility and selection criteria

Adaptation of the model
  Considers local conditions

Figure 9.19. Critical Elements of the HIRe Model

Research on Support Networks

In the United States, the rehabilitation of psychiatrically disabled individuals has recently taken a significant turn. In the last ten years, and proceeding through this decade, deinstitutionalization has taken on serious proportions. Research of the 1950s and 1960s demonstrated the effects of institutionalization on persons with psychotic and affective disorders. In the mid 1970s, alternatives to total institutionalization were promoted for this population. Regional in-patient and out-patient clinics and centres became a popular mode for transferring those with better controlled psychological problems into non-institutionalized settings in which alternative methods for ameliorating psychological problems could be redirected or retrained for later transfer to 'more normal' settings.

In the past decade we have seen major actions taken, essentially to close down virtually all 'institutions for the life long care of persons with permanent mental disabilities'. While the increased rate at which deinstitutionalization is taking place has been goaded on by public deficits, the major impetus for deinstitutionalization has come from the advocacy which followed changes in social attitudes about what are desirable conditions for all citizens: community inclusion, normalization, *and* real competitive employment.

Goals now are to achieve life-conditions for previously institutionalized individuals that are most like those of non-institutional members, while still ensuring their safety and that their disability needs are met. Daytime hours are to include therapeutic and productive activities provided in settings away from the residential setting and in settings where normal work, learning, and recreation occur. There is evidence that people with active psychiatric disabilities can participate productively and, like others with life long and cyclic needs, can work and earn a living when appropriate supports are provided: work schedules may not be the same, how work is arranged may differ, and different forms of on- and off-the-job supports are likely to be needed.

As might be expected, the supports these individuals might require will differ and must be available and accessible as their behaviours and needs change and when the effects of disability reoccur. These needs suggest that access to appropriate case care and rehabilitation under off-job circumstances may be more critical than the behaviour problems that occur because of or during work. How well one controls psychological responses off-the-job might be the greater problem for keeping these individuals employed.

My colleague Karl Botterbusch is attempting to develop a conceptual model for support systems that can be used by consumers and rehabilitation practitioners to guide community development of networks and mechanisms and which can promote individual access and retention of quality employment. The model he is working toward is depicted in Figure 9.20. It suggests that consumers encounter problems or needs in relation to work (loading across the two dimensions on the face of the block) and that solutions to these problems may be derived through training, through behaviours of the individual, and through professional intervention. He proposes that these interactive interventions may increase a capacity or alter an environment. Such capacity acquisition and skills

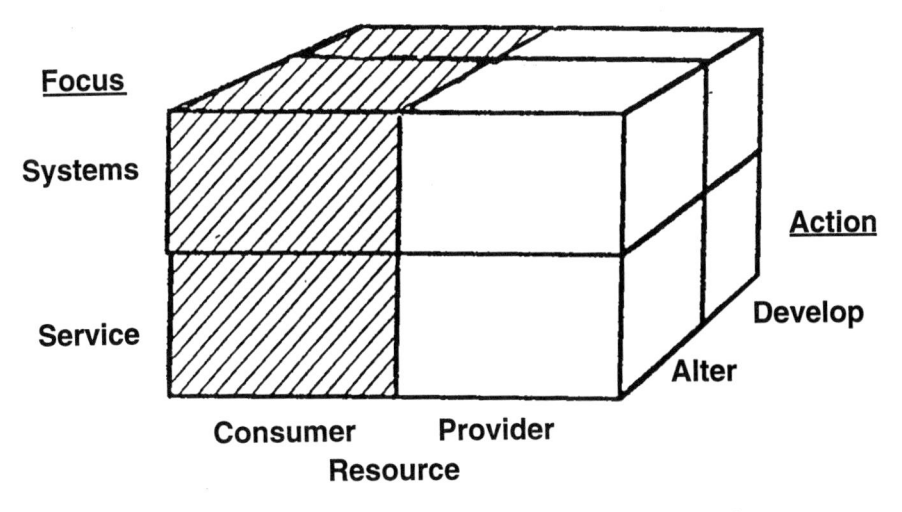

Figure 9.20. Support Systems for Persons with Life Long Rehabilitation Needs

development may be on the part of the rehabilitation consumer or the rehabilitation process.

One hundred and seven individuals in four major midwestern cities participated in a one-hour interview in which they were presented a matrix in which they sequentially identified up to ten problems they were having in retaining employment, the importance of each for them, and the resource they found effective in helping them resolve those problems. Their average age was 36 years, 60 per cent of the subjects were male, 22 per cent were black or hispanic, 35 per cent were unemployed, but ready for placement, and 24, 14, and 27 per cents, respectively, were working in sheltered, enclave, and competitive employment. Of those working competitively or in enclaves, they worked 28 hours per week, were earning $5.21 per hour, and were employed in their present job for nearly a year. Stability of employment and hours worked per week varied widely within the sample, however.

Figure 9.21 depicts the prevalence of problems and how importantly they rated each when the problem was identified (10 was highest importance). With nearly one-half of the individuals seeking community-based employment, it is not surprising that nearly 70 per cent report that their most difficult and important problem is in 'finding and subsequently keeping their job'. Financial woes, what to do with their leisure time, relationships with family members, and how to obtain quality housing are among their top problems: these are problems that are not that atypical for any of us. At first, it is surprising that 'crisis help', 'transportation', 'safety', and 'access to various services' do not appear high on their lists, until we consider that these individuals were located in inner-urban settings with publicly supported transportation and were currently connected with a community facility.

Extent to which problems are identified	Rank	Rated importance
More than a half		
Finding and keeping a job	1	8.80
Financial help	2	8.14
Doing things just for fun	3	6.76
Support from family	4	7.76
Housing	5	8.38
More than one-third		
Medical and dental services	6	7.25
Friendship and intimacy	7	7.11
Getting vocational training	8	7.61
Mental health treatment and therapy	9	7.95
Finding out what services are available	10	6.77
More than a fifth		
Transportation	11	6.88
Protection from danger	12	7.56
More responsive services	13	6.61
Services developed by consumers	14	7.40
Consumer support and self-help groups	15	7.18
Less than a fifth		
Coordinated and organized services	16	6.85
Consumer advocacy	17	6.67
Crisis help and intervention	18	7.35
Other problems	19	8.70

Figure 9.21. Rank Order and Rated Importance of Problems Encountered by 107 Persons with Serious Mental Illness

As one looks through the rankings of most important sources for solving problems, we see on Figure 9.22 some of the reasons why those problems were as low on their lists as they were. Besides identifying themselves (a nice healthy response), many of the most important sources for them (i.e., which are effective in helping them to solve problems) were already people actively involved in their rehabilitation. Parents, special friends, and individuals within a support group were also considered particularly beneficial by them. Given the prevailing emphasis on the 'inherent value of natural supports', it was somewhat surprising to find that people in their wider personal and work environment were not often found to be helpful. These findings suggest at least two possibilities:
- the findings may challenge the concept of 'natural supports' which postulates that structures outside family and rehabilitation can be meaningful sources of continuing support; and/or

Persons most important in solving problems	Most important three ranked
Own Self	1
Rehabilitation Professionals	
Mental Health Case Worker	2
Case Manager at Facility	3
Psychiatrist	6
Other Facility Staff	7
Other Professionals	8
Vocational Rehabilitation Counsellor	10
Medical Doctor	16
Family	
Parents	4
Spouse and Children	12
Brothers and Sisters	13
Personal Environment	
Friends	5
Persons in a Self-Help Group	9
Housing Provider and Staff	11
Religious Leader	14
Neigbours	20
Other	17
Work Environment	
Employer	15
Job Coach	18
Co-workers	19

Figure 9.22. Rankings of Persons Grouped for Solving Problems

- the rehabilitation system/processes may create a dependence on the 'therapeutic' rather than the 'natural' environment which most of us find to be supportive to our sustained involvement and productive lives.

If the first is the case, developmental efforts may need to be directed toward establishing support systems through existing rehabilitation organizations in order to insure the 'life long' access to supports through current community resources: for example, case management provided through psychosocial programmes and/or rehabilitation facilities. Presently, it is not unusual for rehabilitation facilities to provide these types of services for the problems most often identified (e.g., employment, assistance in housing and finance). However, the present rehabilitation configuration does not assure that the individual can have easy access to those services on a crisis basis. The American system requires that a 'case be open' before funds for services can be expended, while need for reaccess may be cyclic and well after the case is typically 'closed and rehabilitated'.

If created dependence is the case, the problem becomes much more complicated with individuals who do, in many respects, have cyclic and, but life long needs for access. The problems they identify are not likely to disappear, though the intensity may change at different times. This may raise what can be a serious ethical dilemma for the professional concerned with future remissions, episodes, or recurrent needs. Whereas established linkages through present services assures greater likelihood of access to needed services, to what degree does such an assurance *prevent or further limit* the individual in their selection of preferred resources that may be instrumental to achieve their rehabilitation goals? Does rehabilitation yield creative user-dependence or does it create a more informed capacity among individuals to choose among the available venues? What does rehabilitation mean among people who will probably always be limited in their potential to participate in society's benefits because of the burden presented by disability and the limits placed by our present technological-professional capacities impact on such disabilities?

Alternative Community-Based Models

Both Thomas's and Botterbusch's work raises questions about what is possible among truly severely affected individuals, given today's technology and today's rehabilitation models. Their research is clear in suggesting that models which are predicated on a 'restore and achieve a rehabated status' do not fit with the disability needs among these individuals. Their research also raise questions as to the applicability of systems (i.e., as used in American rehabilitation) with a prescribed regime built upon models for 'disability groups' with predictable patterns of disability progression, stabilization, and terminal consequences. Among these two 'types of individuals', it appears that we must devise models which successfully account for the wide variability among them at various points in their lives.

If we continue to find that such responses are not highly predictive under current model efforts (a condition necessary when models are developed for groups of individuals), we must begin to give more serious consideration to other alternatives in 'model development'. One such alternative may be to dispense with the assumption that the individuals classified by disability have enough in common (i.e., their etiology, syndromes, constellations) to justify developing generalized models. For individuals of these two types of disabilities, the more acceptable alternative may be to put our efforts into developing generally acceptable practices (both functionally and ethically) and standards of care with which professionals (probably in conjunction with consumers) can reasonably draw upon to deal with the full gamut of behavioural and social consequences that *may occur* during the individual's life when he or she is under greatest control of their disability. This would of course have significant consequences for the preparation of 'qualified professionals' who might be expected to interleave more individual-level strategies and pharmacological-type tools.

Up to this point we have focused as much on intra-disability characteristics and their apparent effects on employment and community integration. Let us for the moment move over to a more direct look at one general format for community-based models: that is, Group Work Models. At the outset, I will share one of my biases about community-based employment. I think community-based employment can provide opportunities for people with severe disabilities to participate in, to become a part of, any nation's broader society and to reap the benefits (and consequences, both positive and negative). As a new set of options, they may provide opportunities not available before (or previously considered affordable). Where community standards deem economic participation of great importance together with work which provides good wages and the use of those wages to acquire basic needs, these models may offer the most appropriate options.

Over a longer perspective of models, we probably need to consider a much more transitive view of the quality of employment models: A transitive view which would allow for:

- various shades and hues of employment
- movement among the options (i.e., from protected, to group, to individual, to competitive employment)

would provide:

- appropriate forms of support
- the social capacities needed to encourage an individual's movement between options
- those supports that assure their rights to make informed choices (in keeping with the individual's interests and abilities)
- those supports that help assure that benefits from such choices are reasonably achieved.

The direction of research in this area is not to demonstrate which model is the best. Rather, it is to show clear models and to find out what it is that each actually provides to consumers and other rehabilitation constituencies. Figure 9.23 suggests some of the dimensions along which our work is proceeding. As examples, we see how an individual benefits (earnings, integration), and the associated costs borne under each model (costs to achieve a desired quality level, investments families might have to make to maintain that level of quality) are jointly considered.

While each of our staff is actively engaged in model development and evaluation research my colleague, Charles Coker is establishing baseline measurements of benefits achieved through various forms of group employment among carefully matched samples of individuals with developmental disabilities. From here, we expect to move to charting similarity of benefits among matched samples of persons in individual supported and competitive employment, to examining the economic consequences for society (e.g., comparative costs of different options); and the design and implementation of the models and on-the-job behaviours were directly observed and verified by project staff; and each subject was interviewed with the Job Satisfaction Interview. This instrument is a highly structured inquiry into the individual's satisfaction with working conditions, opportunities for advancement, nature of supervision and support, and experiences in integration with non-disabled persons. It is a quantified

122 / *VOCATIONAL REHABILITATION AND EUROPE*

Utility Related to Earnings

[Bar chart showing three community-based models A, B, C with four bars each representing Off-Job Support, On-Job Support, Staff Ratio, and Cost]

Community-Based Models

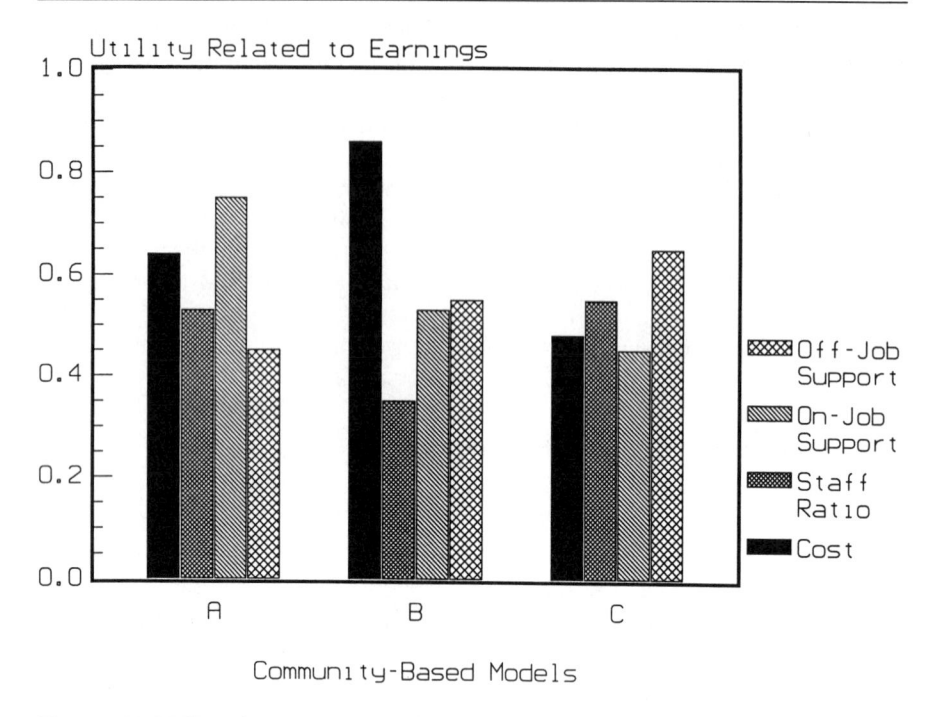

Figure 9.23. Utility of Community-Based Delivery Systems

adaption of a similar interview schedule used by Dr Christine Mason from the National Association of Rehabilitation Facilities in its exemplary practices demonstration project in 1989.

Figures 9.24 and 9.25 reveal some of these comparative findings. The 'internal' group model is sheltered employment, based on who controls the payroll and provides the job supervision. Enclave employment was typically in domestic services and groundskeeping throughout Minneapolis-St Paul, Minnesota. The affirmative industry employed people ready for employment and they were assembling high technology parts. Individuals worked between half-time to three-quarters time (based on an eight-hour workday) on the days they worked. Individuals in sheltered and affirmative jobs worked most steadily, while individuals in enclaves experienced seasonal down time (winter is very long in Minneapolis). With wage rates higher in the affirmative industry and more hours of work available across the year, their gross and net earnings were the highest. Productivity was judged lowest among sheltered employees. Once productivity is taken into account (the lower section of the exhibit), hourly wage differences between shelter and other more integrated forms of employment become more dramatic. One anomaly to note is how differently people in sheltered and in affirmative industries perceive their 'average work day': about one-hour longer than their payroll records indicate. I have no idea what that means, except that it's not unusual for individuals on crews to have to keep track of their actual on-job time and they may include the time they are in transit to the job site in their estimations.

Employment benefit variables	Means for models			Significance of mean differences		
	Internal (a)	Enclave (b)	Affirmative (c)	a–b	a–c	b–c
Totals for year						
Days worked	235.77	169.35	219.64	x	.	x
Hours worked	995.43	998.42	1318.29	.	x	x
Gross wages	1593.82	2684.71	3726.56	x	x	x
Net wages	1365.40	2441.47	3140.35	x	x	x
Productivity	31.36	52.19	52.33	x	x	.
Averages						
Hourly wage	1.56	2.58	2.68	x	x	.
Hours per day	4.25	5.81	5.86	x	x	.
Estimated hourly wage (based on 100 per cent productivity)	4.78	5.05	5.65	.	x	.
Perception hours						
per day	5.61	5.81	6.72	.	x	x

Figure 9.24. *Employment Benefits Under Group Models*

Again, we sought a picture of overall satisfaction and differences between the three models. As you review the right side of Figure 9.25, where tests of significance are summarized, several important findings are revealed: on an 11-item scale of satisfaction, their reported satisfaction was high, and individuals in sheltered workshops were slightly less satisfied than individuals working in enclaves, had multiple jobs over the year, and considered that their next job would be better than the one they presently had. About 30 per cent of sheltered and enclave employees would change jobs if they could. Keep in mind that enclaves are often work that is similar to that which might be done in a sheltered setting. Individuals, under all three models, indicate satisfaction with the socialization and integration available through their jobs: they have adequate opportunity to be with their friends, they perceive opportunity for integration with non-disabled persons as adequate, and reported that their choices to be integrated were positively received.

There are important wage and earnings differences among the group models, yet reported preferences for alternative employment do not seem to appear. None of the employment studied here would provide the individuals with sufficient earnings to live independently. Hourly wages are well blow 'minimum wage scales' and annual earnings are at best 25 to 30 per cent of the poverty level. In disposable income (i.e., net earnings), individuals working outside the sheltered

124 / VOCATIONAL REHABILITATION AND EUROPE

Satisfaction measures Satisfaction measures	Internal (a)	Means for models Enclave (b)	Affirmative (c)	Significance of mean differences a–b a–c b–c
Total job satisfaction	8.64	9.94	9.36	x . .
Demands of job				
Difficultly (Easy/Neither/Difft)	1.68	1.79	1.41	. . .
Boring (Fun/Neither/Boring)	1.46	1.43	1.42	. . .
Future work (Bettr/Same/Wrse)	1.57	1.84	1.70	x . .
Satisfaction with job				
Job pay (Bettr/Same/Wrse)	2.31	2.18	2.15	. . .
Per cent would change job	34.00	25.00	9.09	. x .
Socialization with Friends				
(Three T–F items)	2.84	2.93	2.88	. . .
Integration with Non-Disabled (4 items)				
Opportunity	3.08	3.15	3.17	. . .
Chose to Integrate	3.50	3.80	3.64	. . .
Number Jobs in Last Year	4.77	2.10	3.86	x . .

Figure 9.25. Satisfaction Under Group Models

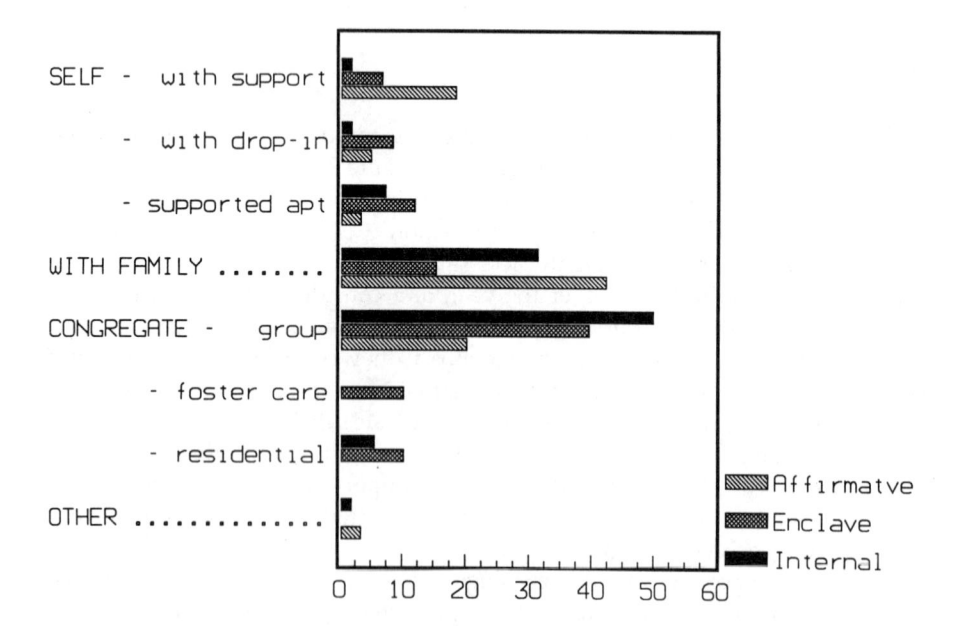

Figure 9.26. Living Arrangements for Group Workers

setting earn between $1000 and $1500 more disposable income (540–810 pounds sterling) per year. Subsidizing for basic needs, for housing, and for on-/off-job support would continue to be highly necessary. As Figure 9.26 indicates, for either disability related problems or because incomes are insufficient to cover real living costs, the large majorities of individuals must live in congregate forms of residences. Only among the affirmative employees did we find 'living by self' to be an option.

As would be expected among samples of individuals with low productivity rates (i.e., between 32 and 52 per cent of the industrial standard), there was a considerable amount of on-job support required, as reported on Figure 27: In doing the job, checking quality, refining skills, in reinforcing, and in helping them to get the job done. Where a job coach was present, the job coach invariably carried out this function. Where the employer's work supervisor was available, that individual typically provided the necessary supervision and training. In essence, these individuals were well aware of what they were being supervised in and knew where to go for assistance in doing or keeping up with the job.

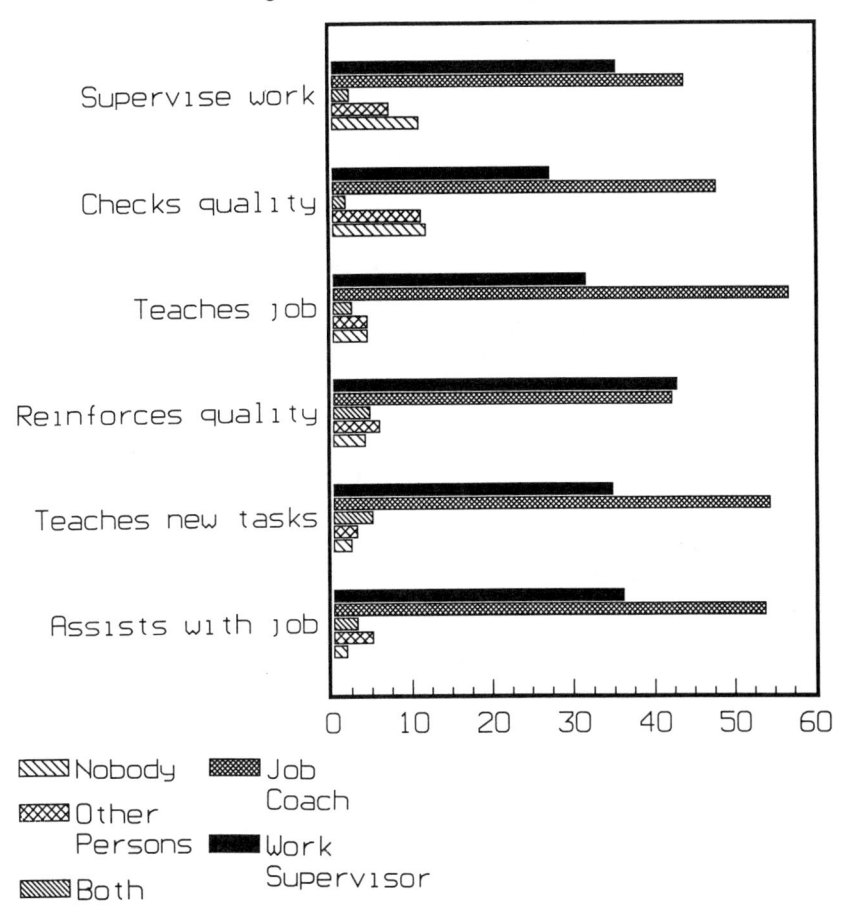

Figure 9.27. Supervision and Support Services (N = 166)

As other researchers are finding, there is not the marked dissatisfaction that might have been expected 'while employed in specific form of employment'. About 95 per cent of workers in enclaves got their job through agency efforts. Friends and the rehabilitation facility were identified by sheltered workers as responsible for getting them the job (32 and 47 per cent, respectively). For those in enclaves, 28 per cent reported that friends and family and 26 per cent reported that the agency found them the job.

What Coker's data does not address, however, is the extent to which personal choice was an essential part of the selecting, getting, and staying with the job. Neither do those data deal with the individual's 'comparative' satisfaction with their work experiences. In other words, these data do not provide information about their informed preferences for one form of employment over another or the consequent satisfaction they may or may not have when they change jobs. Job acquisition patterns among non-disabled persons in this country are greatly influenced by economic conditions and job availability. Job finding is most effective through friends and family and 'choice-need' is more often than not the deciding factor in taking a job or changing jobs. As in the non-disabled workforce, we may find that the 'jobs they left' were not as satisfactory to them as the jobs they now take or that there is something of a penchant for realizing that what was not available to them might make them more discriminating in subsequent job acquisitions.

Community Developed Models

Sometime in the next two years we will share more of the findings from the remainder of our research and development programme on community-based rehabilitation. Perhaps, at that time, we will be together again and share our common experiences and frustrations in building such models. Right now, though, in addition to the research discussed above, we are working with rehabilitation facilities and consumer groups in Wisconsin and Minnesota to help them design, develop, implement, and demonstrate locally appropriate models for serving people with severe disabilities.

As Figure 9.28 simply depicts, through our funds and those from a couple of collaborating agencies, we are presently helping consumers and practitioners design and put into place 11 model programmes. Our research advantage is that we can watch them come of age and have (or

Project Goals:
 Community-Based Employment
 Social Integration
 Consumer Involvement

Processes:
 Consumer Input and Direction
 Technical Assistance
 Facility Designs Model
 Quality Assurance
 Self-Advocacy in Diffusion

Eleven (11) Models Supported:
 Five (5) Traumatic Brain Injury
 Six (6) Serious Mental Illness

Figure 9.28. Support for Development of Community-Derived Models

not have) impact on the earnings and integration of persons with traumatic brain injury and with serious psychiatric disabilities.

Recommendations on Community-Based Models

What does this all mean to us (and, possibly, you as well) as we try to develop and implement models with a strong link to the individual's community? There are some important recommendations (listed on Figure 9.29) that are apparent from the research I have so far talked about. While some of them are especially germane for traumatic brain injury, they probably are also relevant when we think about serving other populations with significant life long disabilities.

Models development
  Inclusion of constitutents in planning
  Range of disabilities
  Models for moderate severity of disability
  Program criteria
  Critical linkages
  Established long-term funding
  Support groups
  Factors essential for success

Use of rehabilitation facilities
  Experience in vocational services in community settings
  Capacity for replacement workers
  Employer contact networks
  Staff trained in relevant vocational disciplines
  Availability to provide training, crisis intervention
  Established linkages with critical constituencies

Barriers to serving persons with traumatic brain injury
  Long-term funding
  Number of qualified professionals with trauma experience
  High turnover
  Inadequate training, opportunities, and experience

Figure 9.29. Recommendations on Developing Community-Based Models

The hard lessons we are coming to grips with are those represented for model development and in the area of barriers. The premises upon which the National Institute is currently attempting to reshape American research policy are not without a credible basis when we are concerned with 'models that work'.

'Academically' imposed models (in the most pejorative sense) do not translate well to real situations nor do they translate well to alternate disability groups. Inclusion of relevant constituencies, awareness of critical linkages, sensitivity to local conditions, compassion in our understanding of individual needs, and an honest appraisal of when and with whom the 'model' *doesn't work*, are essential when we go about building and testing models which we hope to be applicable to real people's needs.

Keeping such models working requires an operational base in the community that can meet certain community-relevant and model-relevant demands: Fiscal responsibility, qualified staffing, interagency linkages, a facility. Maintaining them at levels of quality and of continuing value for individuals with long-term needs requires two fold solutions. We must make substantial progress in finding better ways to fund the non-consumer-wage aspects of these models (e.g., on-/off-job supports, wages for qualified professional personnel to deliver supports). We must solve the challenges presented for the professionals who must work under high stress demands, for low wages, under uncertainty, and with minimal opportunities to develop the skills and experiences upon which they can draw for the variety of strategies which are so typically needed with these individuals.

Pressing Issues of Common Concern in Vocational Rehabilitation Research

Allow me now to draw together from the research and from the broad landscape of American practice and rehabilitation facilities and propose six research priorities (on Figure 9.30) which I believe we must resolve through research and public policy in the coming decade:

(1) Consumer applicable rehabilitation processes. In models development, we must again put an emphasis on rehabilitation processes and those processes in relation to the goals which individuals and our societies wish to pursue. As we look to responding to the needs of persons with increasingly individualized responses to disability, we may need to focus our research efforts on individual treatment strategies. General models and system-usable models may not be appropriate alternatives, given our state of science: research to determine severity, population, and qualitative indicators are needed. There is need for individually-referenced models, as well as group-referenced models.

(2) Research on life long and cyclic rehabilitation needs. We have yet to come up with a meaningful definition of severity. Disability-bound approaches and functional approaches seem to have inherent limitations. Severity may mean life long and/or cyclic needs. Research which significantly track the life experiences and interventions with persons like those we have been talking about today would be most applicable.

(3) Long-term benefits and impacts. What are the consequence of disability and treatment under our 'models'? However we label our models or processes, research needs to help rehabilitation better understand how individuals respond to disability and the quality of impact which defensible processes have on them and on society. Many of the models we now apply have very weak, at best, data to support the value claimed for them among either consumer or rehabilitation constituencies.

Consumer applicable rehabilitation processes
  Severity
  Population
  Qualitative

Life long and cyclic rehabilitation needs
  Access
  Services
  Supports and families
  Economics

Long term benefits and impacts
  Consequences for intended beneficiaries
  Consequences for provider

Public and private sector alternatives
  Delivery
  Supports
  Financing
  Responsibility

Capacity building at community level
  Distinctive rural capacities
  Long-term services
  Planning capacities
  Economic capacities
  Alternative delivery systems for community-based facilities
  Organization structures
  Quality assessment

Human capacities and resources
  Constituencies
  Temporal capacities

Figure 9.30. *Priority Research Issues in 1992*

(4) Public and private alternatives. Likewise, popular and unpopular alternatives need to be given more serious scrutiny. To what extent can certain delivery processes be provided through full cost-recovery and/or through partnerships involving both private and public funding? Are there effective means (via policy, and practice changes) which could shift the delivery of long-term needs (e.g., on-job supports) to non-public funds or sources?

(5) Capacity building at the community level. Capacity building within the community is of special importance in the US system. The ultimate level of delivery is through community agencies, yet significant research has not been entertained to determine how the community-level 'facility' should be organized, staffed, funded, or positioned within the service and business environments.

(6) Human capacities and resources. Quality of services are limited by the availability of appropriately trained professionals and paraprofessionals. Should the community-level provider assume a more significant role in rehabilitation policy, a more vital quality of staff will be required: professionals with high quality skills, staff with capability to renew and redirect their use of skills, and organizations with a renewable human resource.

Lessons To Be Learned

Finally, are there lessons I might share? The European community, as it is now emerging, will change for ever the relationships and international needs among western nations. While nationalism has been well ingrained in our respective consciousnesses, as we begin to see our separate problems more in light of how they are common to the people of our respective nations, the bases for more lasting solutions to issues of humanity, equity, and quality of life achieved by persons throughout our two hemispheres will be available. Economically, politically, and socially nations are coming to resemble each other more closely, I suspect. Our needs in some areas are probably more similar now than any of us might ever have expected: for example, the level of burden we all bear for national health care; the needs each of our nations have to retain a strong employment base for our citizens; the needs we each have to solve rehabilitation and economic problems arising as our most severely disabled citizens no longer die in large numbers, but reach maturity and can be a part of our national lives through the 20, 30, and 40 years of their productive lives.

The main lesson I believe we have learned is that some of the problems we need to address through research may no longer be as idiographic to a given nation's economic and political system as was the case before these changes took place. Now, we may come to find that the solutions to serious rehabilitation problems may be more generalizable: the solutions to depression arrived at through research in Berlin can work in Barcelona; the treatment strategies demonstrated with alcoholics in Lucerne may be adapted to our friends in Dublin; the behavioural control processes found effective with selected syndromes among traumatically brain-injured persons in agricultural Afghanistan may be replicable in rural Montana; the assessment procedures derived in Amsterdam may after all work with New York's psychiatric population.

My nation is pursuing an elusive goal in rehabilitation. We are trying to change nationally how people with disabilities are seen and responded to, and the extent to which they are afforded access to virtually every sector of American life. The nations you represent here are pursuing an elusive goal of cross-national unification. As we both pursue these goals, they offer exciting opportunities and perils, especially, to the 'way things always were'. It may be that the issues of vocational rehabilitation are now a territory on which we may find real opportunities to achieve, more efficiently and meaningfully, less culturally limited understandings of serious disabilities and of the options that can creatively add to the quality of the lives of these individuals.

References

Graves, W.H. (1991) Participatory Action Research: A new paradigm for disability and rehabilitation research. Paper presented to the Annual Meeting of the National Association of Rehabilitation Research and Training Center, at Washington, DC, on 7 May 1991.

Working Definitions

Consumers

These are individuals directly affected by disability (the individual with the impairment, the care-giver) and persons less directly affected by disabilities (close friends, family, co-workers). They include, therefore, those individuals who are expected to benefit in some way from the rehabilitation practices we promote. They do not, in this context, include people who make use of research (i.e., professionals, policy-makers).

Rehabilitation constituencies

These are the individuals, organizations, and groups involved in rehabilitation, but not the immediate or secondary beneficiaries of the rehabilitation process. These include the professionals providing a part of the rehabilitation service, the agency paying for a service, the employer adapting to an individual's needs, the advocate attempting to affect public policy, the federal agency funding research or services, the US Congress.

Rehabilitation facility

A legally constituted organization which provides identifiable rehabilitation processes with articulate rehabilitation goals for both the consumer and such other constituencies that may purchase its services. While it may provide long-term care (medical, residential) or protected employment, its primary purpose is to achieve acceptable outcomes and uses rehabilitation professionals and paraprofessionals to work with individuals to achieve stated outcomes.

Community-based rehabilitation

Rehabilitation processes provided in the most normal setting appropriate to the maturity of current practices and technology and the desires and capacities of the individual consumer. Rehabilitation goals are identified and pursued. Community-based employment, supported employment, supported living, independent living, community-based assessment, on-job skills training, behavioural-vocational adjustment are all included under this generic term, but the term itself makes no social statement about hours, wages, nature of activity, preference for the activity.

Contributors

Elizabeth Chennell is a freelance writer and editor.

Dr Frank Coffield is Professor of Education at the University of Durham.

Dr Paul Cornes is Director of Eurorehab Services.

Dr Michael Floyd is a Reader in the Department of Systems Science at City University and Director of its Rehabilitation Resource Centre.

Katherine Floyd is a Lecturer at the School of Tropical Medicine at the University of Liverpool.

Dr Donal McAnaney is Director of Development for Rehab, the leading provider of vocational rehabilitation services in Ireland. He is also Director of a Masters programme in Social and Vocational Rehabilitation at University College, Dublin.

Dr Fred Menz is a Director of Research in the Stout Vocational Rehabilitation Institute at the University of Wisconsin.

Adam Pozner is a researcher at OUTSET.

Dr Erwin Seyfried is Director of a Research Unit at the FHVR in Berlin, concerned with vocational training, the labour market and evaluation.